SOMATIC EXERCISES FOR BEGINNERS

The Complete Illustrated Step-by-Step Guide to Lose Weight, Eliminate Chronic Pain, Anxiety, and Stress | Included 30-Day Workout Plan"

BY

AVA STERLING

© Copyright 2024 (Ava Sterling) all rights reserved.

This document is geared towards providing exact and reliable information with regard to the topic and issue covered. The publication is sold with the idea that the publisher is not required to render accounting, officially permitted, or otherwise qualified services. If advice is necessary, legal or professional, a practiced individual in the profession should be ordered.

From a Declaration of Principles which was accepted and approved equally by a Committee of the American Bar Association and a Committee of Publishers and Associations.

In no way is it legal to reproduce, duplicate, or transmit any part of this document in either electronic means or in printed format. Recording of this publication is strictly prohibited, and any storage of this document is not allowed unless with written permission from the publisher. All rights reserved.

The information provided herein is stated to be truthful and consistent, in that any liability, in terms of inattention or otherwise, by any usage or abuse of any policies, processes, or directions contained within is the solitary and utter responsibility of the recipient reader. Under no circumstances will any legal responsibility or blame be held against the publisher for any reparation, damages, or monetary loss due to the information herein, either directly or indirectly.

TABLE OF CONTENTS

Introduction 7

Chapter 1: History and Origins of Somatic Exercises 8

Chapter 2: Basic Principles and Benefits 10

Chapter 3: Differences Between Somatic and Other Movement Practices 13

Chapter 4: Overcoming Challenges and Frustrations: Setting Realistic Goals and Expectations 14

Chapter 5: Creating an Adequate Space for Practice 16

Chapter 6: Recommended Clothing and Equipment 18

Chapter 7: Mental and Physical Preparation 19

    Physical preparation 19

    Mental preparation 19

Chapter 8: Exercises 21

    Exercises for losing weight 21

        Utkatasana 21

        Bhujangasana or Cobra Pose 22

        Boat Pose 23

        Hip Circles 24

        Leg Circles 26

    Exercises to relieve stress and anxiety 28

        Child Pose 28

        Legs to the wall 29

        Box Breathing 30

- Relaxing circle exercise 31
- Tree Pose 32
- The movement of the Flowing River 34
- The 5-4-3-2-1 Grounding Technique 35
- Butterfly hug 37
- Fish Pose 38
- Corpse Pose 39
- Mountain Pose 41

Exercises for flexibility and stretch 43
- Feldenkrais Thoracic rotation 43
- The Saw 44
- Mermaid 45
- Forward Fold 46
- Eagle Pose 48
- Cow Pose 49
- Spine Stretch Forward 50
- Arm Swings 52
- Single Leg Stretch 53
- Raised arm Pose 55
- Hip opener stretch 56
- Crescent Moon Pose 57

Exercises to calm nervous system 60
- Heaviness exercise 60
- Diaphragmatic breathing or abdominal breathing 61
- The Ujjayi breath 62
- Supta Baddha Konasana 63
- Cat Cow Pose 64

- Erected Pole (zhan zhuang) 65
- Conscious breathing 67
- The position of intoxicating bliss 68
- Exercises to relieve chronic pain 70
  - Pelvic Clock 70
  - Cross twist position 71
  - Garland Pose 72
  - Swan dive 74

Chapter 9: 30-days Somatic Exercises Challenge 76

Conclusions 82

Introduction

Somatic exercises are specific exercises that are often included in somatic therapies, that is, those therapies that focus on the connection between mind and body. Somatic exercises are exercises focused on specific movements that help release tension on a physical level to improve overall well-being.

Somatic exercises are very practical and accessible to anyone, even beginners since they do not require the use of specific equipment or particular skills to perform them.

This book invites you to explore the wealth found within the confines of our bodies by engaging in somatic exercises. A guide that intends to lead you through an inner journey, a path of exploration and reconnection with your bodily dimension.

Somatic exercises represent a bridge to body awareness, an intimate language that will allow you to listen to the stories your body tells, understand the signals it sends you and welcome the wisdom that resides in every muscle, joint and cell.

Through the practice of targeted exercises and awareness of breathing, you will immerse yourself in an unexplored territory, where emotions, tensions and joys are hidden and, indeed, somatized, by our body.

This book aims to be a map for this journey, offering practical tools, reflections and practical advice that will lead you to rediscover the joy of conscious movement, the strength of anchoring in the present and the freedom that comes from bodily awareness.

You will also find targeted exercises that will not only help you reconnect your mind and body but will also help you improve your fitness and flexibility. All the exercises will be explained to you step-by-step; they will be divided into categories, and all the benefits that each single exercise brings to your body will also be listed.

Chapter 1: History and Origins of Somatic Exercises

Somatics, from which somatic exercises derive, is a movement that emphasizes awareness and bodily perception starting from our inside.

One of the key early precursors of the somatic movement in Western culture was the physical culture movement which peaked in the 19th century. This movement represented a significant paradigm shift in the approach to physical health and well-being, seeking to integrate a series of movement practices, known as "gymnastics", within a broader context that included military preparation, athletic activities, medical treatments and even elements from dancing.

The legacy of the 19th century physical culture movement is still evident today. Many of the key concepts such as the importance of physical activity, the connection between mind and body, and the holistic approach to health have been incorporated into modern somatic practices. The evolution of these ideas over time has led to the creation of methods such as the Pilates Method, which draws inspiration from gymnastics and integrates principles of body awareness.

In the 19th century, many physical culture practices were introduced to the United States, influencing how American society viewed exercise and health. Interest in gymnastics and physical culture grew alongside increasing urbanization and industrialization, with a greater awareness of the need to maintain good physical health in a context that also included rapid social changes.

In this context Genevieve Stebbins was one of the key figures in the evolution of physical culture practices in the United States. She was an innovator who developed her own system focused on the integration of physical exercises, breathing and developing inner strength. Her approach integrated elements of gymnastics, dance and yoga.

Many of Genevieve Stebbins' followers, having assimilated her system in the United States, returned to Europe, bringing with them their new ideas about physical culture. This diffusion helped shape the landscape of somatic practices in Europe, giving rise to new approaches and influencing key figures in the evolution of the somatic movement.

Among Genevieve Stebbins' followers who returned to Europe, Elsa Gindler emerged as one of the most significant figures. She, in turn, became an early somatic innovator. Gindler developed his approach to physical culture, placing a strong emphasis on body awareness, breathing, and mind-body integration. Her work had a lasting impact on the formation of European somatic practices and contributed to the development of approaches such as the Gindler Method.

In the 1970s, Thomas Hanna coined the term somatic practices, which included and described a series of physical and mental techniques that all had in common the aim of helping people have greater body awareness through movement and relaxation practices.

Over the past few decades, the field of somatic has experienced significant growth, expanding its influence across diverse disciplines and industries. New incorporations include dance forms such as contact improvisation and Skinner's release technique, along with the application of somatic in therapeutic, occupational, psychological and educational contexts.

The Skinner Release Technique was developed by Joan Skinner as an approach to contemporary dance. This technique focuses on breathing awareness, releasing muscle tension, and facilitating fluid movements through recognition and awareness of body habits. This technique has been integrated into the field of somatic due to its emphasis on tension release and body awareness. The practice aims to improve freedom of movement, reduce pain and promote well-being through active listening to the body.

Somatic exercises are therefore a set of practices that involve body awareness, movement and breathing to improve physical and mental health. These exercises have deep roots in human history and have been developed in different cultures and traditions over time.

Chapter 2: Basic Principles and Benefits

Somatic exercises are a set of exercises that have been created and developed with the aim of improving body awareness, so that we have a deep connection and understanding of how our muscles act and move.

These exercises, therefore, are based on mind-body connection techniques, which aim to accentuate the link between sensation on a physical level and emotional states. What happens outside and how you feel after certain events in your life profoundly affect the way your mind reacts to these events, causing dysfunction even on an organic level. Somatic exercises will help you understand what these tensions are and where they come from and will help you dissolve them through movement.

The basic principle of somatic exercises is, therefore, to improve communication between the muscles and the brain. The slow, gentle movements that are used in these exercises help people tone muscles and improve mobility and overall body movement patterns. By focusing on the sensory receptors located in our muscles, these exercises help us become aware of ourselves and any muscle tension or physical discomfort.

Some examples of somatic exercises include:

- Yoga: A thousand-year-old practice that combines physical postures, breathing and meditation to improve strength, flexibility and body awareness.
- Pilates: A system of exercises that aims to strengthen core muscles, improve posture and promote flexibility through controlled movements.
- Tai chi: An ancient form of Chinese exercise involving slow, fluid, coordinated movements aimed at improving balance, strength and inner calm.
- Feldenkrais: A practice that is based on learning through movement, focusing on body awareness and movement efficiency.
- Alexander Technique: A technique that aims to improve posture and movement through awareness and correction of poor postural habits.
- Mindful Movement: An approach that incorporates present moment awareness while performing physical activities, such as walking, running, or exercising.

These exercises are often used during rehabilitation therapies for those who especially suffer from chronic pain or for rehabilitation after an injury. Furthermore, it has been shown that these types of exercises are very useful for alleviating the discomfort you feel when you are too stressed or suffer from anxiety.

Another benefit of these exercises is that they restore our nervous system, stimulating the responses of the parasympathetic nervous system, which is responsible for the rest and relaxation phases of our body. In this way it will be possible to release any type of physical or mental stress that is stored in our body.

Somatic exercises are also very useful for healing any trauma, be it physical or emotional. In this case, the exercises focus on how past negative experiences are stored in our body and then become a problem on a somatic level as well.

Other benefits of practicing somatic exercises include:

- Sleep problems: Somatic exercises can promote muscle relaxation and reduce tension, helping to improve the quality of sleep.
- Gut problems: By reducing stress and muscle tension, somatic exercises can help improve gut function and reduce symptoms associated with gastrointestinal disorders.
- Chest pain: By working on body awareness and breathing, somatic exercises can relieve muscle tension in the chest area, reducing chest pain.
- Constant Fatigue: By improving posture and stress management, somatic exercises can help reduce chronic fatigue.
- Brain Fog: By improving the mind-body connection and reducing muscle tension, somatic exercises can promote mental clarity and concentration.
- Chronic Muscle Tension: Somatic exercises focus on releasing muscle tension through mindful movement and relaxation, reducing chronic tension.
- The inability to lose weight (especially in the belly): By reducing stress and tension, somatic exercises can help regulate metabolic processes and improve digestion, facilitating weight loss.
- Neck, shoulder and jaw pain: Somatic exercises can help relax stiff muscles and improve posture, reducing pain in these areas.
- Nighttime Teeth Grinding: By improving stress management and reducing muscle tension, somatic exercises can help reduce nighttime teeth grinding.
- Chronic tension headache: By reducing muscle tension and improving posture, somatic exercises can help prevent and reduce chronic tension headaches.
- Difficulty taking full breaths: Somatic exercises can teach you to breathe more fully and consciously, improving your breathing capacity and reducing feelings of shortness of breath.
- Panic Attacks: By promoting relaxation and body awareness, somatic exercises can be helpful in managing panic attacks and reducing their frequency and intensity.

- Bad posture: Somatic exercises can help correct posture through relaxation and realignment of muscles, improving balance and mobility.

Chapter 3: Differences Between Somatic and Other Movement Practices

The main difference between traditional exercises, which focus on the development of strength, muscle mass or flexibility, and somatic exercises, is that the latter shifts this focus to the connection between mind and body, consequently improving our corporeal awareness.

Their main difference compared to other types of exercise therefore lies in the approach centered on sensory experience and body awareness. Somatic exercises focus on listening to the body, awareness of movements and releasing accumulated tensions.

Instead of just focusing on the physical aspect of exercise, such as strength or cardiovascular training, somatic exercises seek to connect with bodily sensations and address any blockages or tension through slow, controlled, and mindful movements. This approach can help release chronic muscle tension and improve posture.

To be more precise, here are the main differences between traditional exercises and somatic exercises:

- Body Awareness: Somatic exercises place a strong emphasis on body awareness. This means that during the exercise you are focused on the sensations and movements of the body, developing a greater mind-body connection. Traditional exercises can focus more on physical performance without necessarily encouraging mindfulness.

- Slower, more controlled movements: Somatic exercises often involve slow, controlled movements that aim to improve movement precision and reduce muscle tension. Traditional exercises can include a variety of intensities and movement styles, with the goal of developing strength, endurance and flexibility.

- Holistic Approach: Somatic exercises often take a holistic approach, viewing the body as an integrated system. This may include awareness of breathing, posture and balance. Traditional exercises can focus on more specific goals such as muscle strengthening, weight loss, or improving athletic performance.

- Engaging the mind: Somatic exercises often incorporate practices that engage the mind, such as meditation or visualization, to improve body awareness. In traditional exercises, the mind may be primarily involved in achieving specific physical goals.

- Adaptability: Somatic exercises can be adapted to suit each practitioner's individual needs and abilities. Traditional exercises can be more structured and focused on predetermined routines.

Chapter 4: Overcoming Challenges and Frustrations: Setting Realistic Goals and Expectations

Dealing with challenges and frustrations while engaging in somatic exercises requires the ability to set both goals and realistic expectations, so as not to fall into frustration and give up immediately before even starting.

Here are some tips for managing frustration:

- Understanding your goals is the first fundamental step to establishing an effective path in somatic exercises. Clearly defining your goals will assist you in staying motivated and evaluating the feasibility of your expectations.
- Be realistic. Setting achievable and realistic goals is essential to maintaining motivation and preventing frustration. Take into consideration your current fitness level, your physical limitations, and the time you can dedicate to somatic exercises when setting goals.
- Evaluate your present level of fitness, taking into account your familiarity and experience with somatic exercises. If you're a beginner, you may want to start with more modest goals and gradually increase them as you gain more confidence and strength.
- Consider your physical limitations. Pay attention to your physical limitations, such as pre-existing injuries, medical conditions, or mobility limitations. Set goals that take these limitations into account and can be adapted to your individual needs.
- Choose measurable, specific goal. Rather than setting vague goals like "improve my fitness," opt for measurable, specific goals like "increase my flexibility" or "maintain a somatic exercise practice for at least X days a week."
- Exercise patience and adopt a gradual approach. Keep in mind that progress may require time and avoid expecting instant outcomes. Choose goals that can be achieved through small, progressive steps and celebrate every success along the way.
- Review and adjust goals as necessary. Regularly revisit your objectives and evaluate their feasibility considering your progress and current situation. Modify your goals if needed to ensure they remain attainable and inspiring.
- Focus on the process, not just the results. Focus on the actions you can control when practicing somatic exercises, such as your form, your breathing, and your body awareness.
- Practice self-kindness. Avoid criticizing yourself harshly if you encounter difficulties or if results don't come immediately. Be kind to yourself and appreciate the progress, even if it's small.

- Work on improving your technique, body awareness, and releasing muscle tension during exercises, rather than focusing solely on external results like weight loss or flexibility.

Chapter 5: Creating an Adequate Space for Practice

Somatic Exercises, as we have seen, are focused on developing body awareness and the mind-body connection. Choosing the right environment to practice such exercises can certainly influence the overall experience and the benefits that follow.

The somatic exercises were created and developed to be practiced in a simple and accessible way for anyone. Since it does not require the use of expensive equipment or specific requirements, practicing these exercises can be performed practically anywhere.

Here are some practical tips on how to create adequate space for your training routine:

- First, look for a quiet place without external distractions. Silence can promote greater concentration on your bodily and mental experience. A quiet environment is essential to promote concentration and connection with movements during Somatic Exercises. Tranquility allows you to reduce external distractions, allowing greater awareness of your body and sensations. Interruptions or unwanted noises can interrupt the flow of awareness and detract from the experience. Additionally, a quiet space can promote deeper relaxation, helping to reduce stress and improve the quality of the somatic experience.

- Make sure the environment where you practice your exercises is well lit so that you can move safely and clearly see what you are doing. Natural light can provide significant advantages, yet it's essential to ensure you also have sufficient artificial lighting.

- Ensure that you have ample room for unrestricted movement. Somatic exercises often involve slow, mindful movements, so avoid crowded or cramped areas of your home.

- Select a setting that induces a sense of comfort for you. It may be helpful to use a mat or soft surface if the exercises require you to sit on the floor. The mat provides some cushioning for the body, making exercises more comfortable. The mat can act as extra support for your joints, offering a soft surface that can help reduce stress on your knees, elbows and other areas of your body during exercises. Many mats are also designed with non-slip surfaces, which is especially useful during dynamic movements or when adopting a stable posture. This helps maintain stability and safety during practice.

- A private environment is ideal for practicing these types of exercises, but if you share the space, let others know you are practicing and kindly ask them to respect your privacy throughout the training session.

- If possible, choose an outdoor location or setting with a window or balcony with a relaxing panoramic view. Nature can help create a peaceful atmosphere and facilitate connection with your body.

Chapter 6: Recommended Clothing and Equipment

The choice of clothes during the practice of Somatic Exercises is an important element in guaranteeing the right comfort and the right freedom of movement.

Wearing loose, comfortable clothing offers several benefits:

- Freedom of movement: Loose clothing allows the body to move freely without restrictions. This is especially important when engaging in exercises requiring prolonged joint mobility or push-ups. Doing so enables your body to naturally adjust to the movements involved in the exercise.
- Body awareness: Wearing comfortable clothes helps maintain greater body awareness. Feeling the body without constraints can facilitate the mind-body connection and improve the perception of physical sensations during practice.
- Relaxation: Loose clothing can help create a relaxed environment. The sensation of comfort promotes muscle relaxation, allowing the body to respond more fluidly to exercises.
- Breathability: Lightweight and breathable fabrics are ideal for avoiding overheating during physical activity. Maintaining an adequate body temperature can contribute to a more pleasant and comfortable practice.
- Ease of execution: Wearing comfortable clothes makes it easier to perform the exercises, especially if they require delicate movements or specific positions.

As far as material goes, stretchy fabrics like cotton or breathable materials work well. Stretch fabrics allow for greater flexibility and adaptability to body movements. This flexibility is particularly advantageous for exercises that require extensive ranges of motion.

The breathable fabrics allow good ventilation during physical activity. This is essential to maintain your comfort and prevent overheating by keeping you cool and dry. Cotton can absorb moisture, helping to keep your skin dry during practice. This is important for comfort and can help prevent skin irritation.

Finally, consider practicing barefoot or wearing socks with good traction. Going barefoot or wearing socks with good traction allows for a greater connection with the ground. This can improve body awareness and perception of sensations during exercises, contributing to a deeper and more conscious practice.

Additionally, without rigid shoes or footwear limitations, the foot can move more naturally, improving flexibility and mobility.

Chapter 7: Mental and Physical Preparation

The primary objective of somatic practices is to resolve traumas and tensions, physical and mental. For this reason, the most important thing to do during the exercises is to focus on releasing all negative feelings and thoughts. For this reason, the initial step is to establish a predetermined and specific goal. Having a goal will help you tackle individual exercises with the right mentality and with the correct approach. In this way you will also be more encouraged to practice the exercises more consistently and obtain greater results.

The other fundamental step is relaxation. Regardless of what you want to achieve from the exercises, relaxing both your body and mind is a key part of completely transforming your physical and mental health.

Physical preparation

with a gentle warm-up to prime your body for the upcoming movements. You might engage in joint mobilization exercises or focus on deep breathing to enhance blood circulation.

Incorporate dynamic stretching to improve flexibility and prepare muscles for movement. Examples may include joint rotation movements or controlled stretching exercises.

Maintain correct posture during preparation and exercises. Proper posture promotes proper body alignment and can help prevent injuries.

Gradually increase the intensity of the exercises. Start with simpler movements to allow your body to adapt before moving on to more advanced exercises.

Pay attention to bodily sensations while preparing. If you feel pain or discomfort, adapt your exercises accordingly and don't push your body beyond its limits. One of the critical elements of somatic exercises involves paying close attention to the signals your body is sending. Be aware of physical sensations, muscle tension and movement limitations as you perform the exercises. Respect your body's limits and never force movements beyond your comfort.

Ensure to incorporate sufficient recovery periods into your exercise routine to enable your body to recuperate effectively from somatic exercises. Rest is essential for muscle growth, tissue repair and injury prevention.

Mental preparation

Place an emphasis on being aware of the physical sensations that arise during somatic exercises. Observe muscle tension, sensations of stretching and releasing, and changes in muscle tone.

Use mindfulness as a tool to increase awareness of bodily sensations during somatic exercises. Concentrate on the present moment without passing judgment, allowing sensations to arise and flow naturally. Center your attention on your internal sensations, setting aside worries, distractions, and irrelevant thoughts. Direct your focus towards the movements you're executing and the sensations arising within your body.

Practice acceptance and refrain from judgment towards yourself and your emotions throughout somatic exercises. Embrace your body as it is in that moment, releasing any expectations or desires for specific outcomes. Be kind to yourself and avoid self-criticism.

Mentally visualize yourself performing the somatic exercises with ease, fluidity, and gratitude. Imagine the harmonious flow of movements and the release of muscle tension. This positive visualization can help you mentally prepare and improve your performance during practice.

Practice gratitude for your body and participation in somatic exercises. Recognize the value of taking care of yourself through mindful practice and thank your body for its strength, flexibility and resilience.

After practice, take time to recover mentally and physically. Reflect on your experience, the sensations you experienced and any teachings you received. This recovery and reflection phase is essential for integrating the effects of somatic exercises into your daily life.

Chapter 8: Exercises

In this chapter you will find a series of 40 somatic exercises, designed to improve your physical and mental well-being. This collection of exercises offers a wide range of easy-to-perform movements, designed to help you lose weight, relieve stress, anxiety, improve flexibility and strength, as well as calm the nervous system. Furthermore, you will also find specific exercises to relieve chronic pain, offering a holistic solution to improve your overall health and well-being.

Each exercise is accompanied by a brief description and the benefits it can bring to your body and mind.

Exercises for losing weight

Losing weight may be a challenge, but it's a feasible objective for numerous individuals. Alongside a well-rounded diet, engaging in regular physical activity is essential for reaching and sustaining a desirable weight. Somatic exercises offer a holistic approach that involves mind and body to promote weight loss in a healthy and sustainable way.

Utkatasana

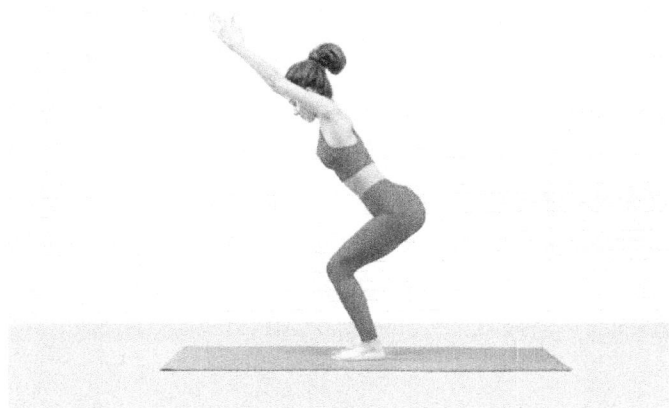

Also known as "chair yoga," it is a standing position that involves the legs, arms and torso. It is an exercise that involves the use of key muscles of the body and can be included in a somatic practice that serves to contribute to weight loss.

Benefits:
- Utkatasana involves actively activating the core muscles, including the abdominals and lower back muscles. Strengthening the core can lead to better posture and enhanced muscle equilibrium. The chair pose engages

the legs, especially the quadriceps muscles. Working these muscle groups can increase calorie expenditure and contribute to muscle strengthening.

- When performed dynamically and with rhythm, the chair pose can increase the heart rate, thus contributing to a form of light aerobic exercise.

Execution

1. Stand with your heels together and your big toes touching. Lift your toes, opening them like a fan and rest them again to create a wider and more solid base of support.
2. If you have trouble feeling your ankles too close together, move your heels apart, but always keep your big toes parallel. Distribute your body weight evenly across your toes, heels, and both feet until you feel stable.
3. As you exhale, lower your buttocks back and down as if you're preparing to sit on a chair. Place your hands on your thighs. To perform the bend correctly, lift your toes to keep your heels on the ground.
4. Keep your back straight and, especially the lumbar curve, pushing the navel towards the spine.
5. Ensure that your knees are aligned and don't extend beyond your toes.
6. Raise your arms upwards, keeping them parallel to each other. Keep your gaze fixed straight ahead.
7. Remain still in this position and breathe regularly, until your body feels stable and comfortable.
8. To exit the position, inhale, slowly straighten your knees and exhale, lower your arms along your body.

Bhujangasana or Cobra Pose

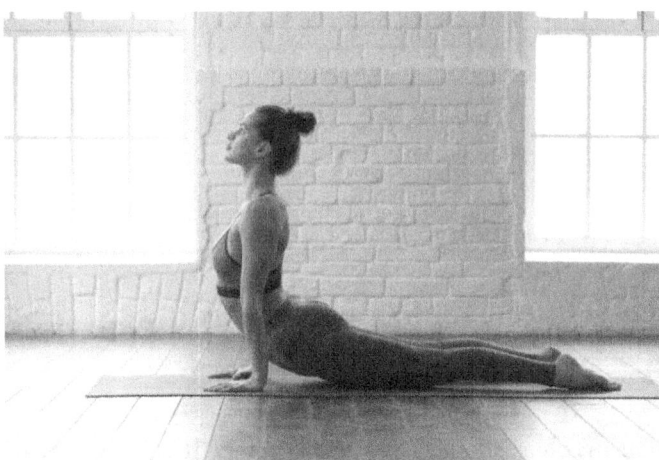

The cobra position is one of the yoga poses that involves an extension of the spine, an opening of the chest and a stretching of the abdominal muscles.

Benefits:

- The cobra pose involves gentle compression of the abdominal organs, which can promote better digestion and proper functioning of the digestive system.

- The cobra pose works several muscle groups, including the muscles of the back, arms and abdomen. Toned muscles can contribute to a more efficient metabolism, potentially aiding weight loss.

Executions:

1. Position yourself on your yoga mat with your stomach facing down.
2. Extend your legs and bring them together, with the instep in contact with the floor.
3. Position your hands on the ground beneath your shoulders, keeping your fingers spread open and pointing forward. Make sure that your hands are placed slightly below your shoulders, maintaining a slight bend in your elbows.
4. Keep your arms bent so that your palms are completely on the ground.
5. Distribute your weight evenly across both hands, creating a stable base.
6. Relax the muscles of your body, focusing on the sensation of opening your chest.
7. Activate your thigh muscles, contract your glutes and lengthen your legs to maintain a solid, stable position.
8. Inhale deeply and, using the muscles of your upper back, arch your trunk, lifting your torso off the ground.
9. Be careful not to push too hard with your hands; try to use your core strength to lift yourself up.
10. Extend your neck and lift your head, keeping your gaze facing forward or slightly upward.
11. Keep your shoulders relaxed and don't lift your shoulder blades too much, trying to maintain a natural alignment of the spine.
12. Maintain regular, deep breathing while in the position.
13. Try to keep your diaphragm open to maximize air flow into your lungs.
14. Hold cobra pose for at least two deep breaths, enjoying the sensation of opening in your chest and front of your body.
15. Exhale slowly and, with control, lower your torso to the ground, returning to the starting position.

Boat Pose

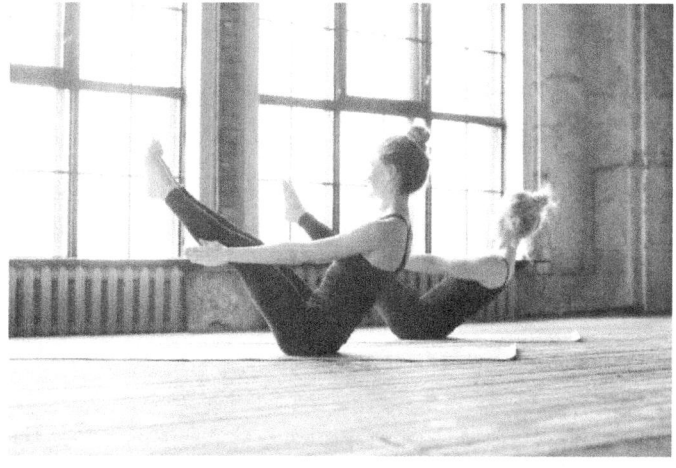

Paripurna Navasana, commonly known as the "full boat pose" in yoga, is a pose that involves lifting the legs and torso, creating a "V" shape with the body.

Benefits:

- The position requires significant effort from the abdominal muscles to keep the body in balance. Engaging in this practice can assist in toning and strengthening your abdominal muscles, leading to improved muscle definition.
- Raising your legs from a sitting position requires the use of your leg muscles, including your quadriceps and hip flexor muscles. Engaging in this exercise can contribute to enhancing muscle strength and endurance in the legs.
- Light compression of the abdominal organs during Paripurna Navasana can promote better digestion and stimulate the functioning of the digestive system, which is important for weight management.
- Exercises that involve multiple muscle groups, such as Paripurna Navasana, can aid in boosting your metabolism. A more active metabolism can aid in the process of burning calories and managing body weight.
- Yoga practice in general, including Paripurna Navasana, can increase body awareness. Being mindful of this fact can prompt individuals to make healthier choices regarding their nutrition and lifestyle, indirectly supporting weight loss efforts.

Execution:

1. Begin in a seated position, with your knees bent at a right angle, thighs parallel to the ground, and feet planted firmly on the floor, hip-width apart.
2. Keep your hands around your thighs, near your knees.
3. Lean your torso backwards, at a right angle to your thighs without collapsing your chest or abdomen.
4. Extend from the tailbone to the top of the head. Activate your abdominal muscles by contracting them inwards. Activate your abdomen, lift your rib cage and stabilize your shoulder blades by bringing them together.
5. Maintain your focus on a specific point ahead of you as you lift your feet off the ground. Continue raising your feet until you can sustain a straight spine and keep your chest lifted. The full position has your legs extended straight at 45 degrees off the ground, with your arms parallel to the ground and your chest raised.
6. Hold the position for several breaths until you feel stable. If you lose your balance, repeat the previous steps and return to the position.
7. To exit the position, gradually bend your knees and return your feet to the ground. Sit with your spine straight and legs crossed, in a simple position.

Hip Circles

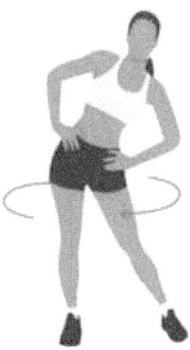

With this exercise that works all the muscles you will have slim thighs and defined abs, as well as more toned shoulders and chest.

Benefits:
- The abdomen is stressed intensely: thanks to the continuous contraction of the powerhouse, in fact, you must stabilize the body while carrying out the movements with your legs, which unbalance you. By keeping your legs tense and raised, you tone your thigh muscles (especially the quadriceps and hip flexors), while the need to support your torso activates your pectorals and deltoids.
- Incorporating hip circles into your workout regimen can enhance body awareness and posture. Maintaining a flexible hip can positively influence the overall alignment of the body.
- Performing hip circles requires concentration and awareness of body movement. This can help develop greater body awareness, which is useful in various physical activities.

Execution:
1. Begin by standing with your feet spaced shoulder-width apart.
2. Keep an upright posture, ensuring your shoulders are relaxed and your weight is evenly distributed on both feet.
3. Begin to move your hips forward, bringing them towards the right side.
4. Continue the movement by bringing your hips back, then to the left side and forward again, creating a circular motion. Visualize tracing a circle with your hips. Execute this movement smoothly and with control.
5. After completing a few clockwise circles, change direction. Shift your hips to the left, then backward, to the right, and forward once more.
6. Keep the movement concentrated in the hip area, avoiding excessive movement in the upper body.
7. You can slightly bend your knees to make the movement easier, but make sure you maintain stability in your lower body.

8. Synchronize the movement of the hip circles with your breathing. For example, inhale as you move your hips forward and exhale as you move them back.

Leg Circles

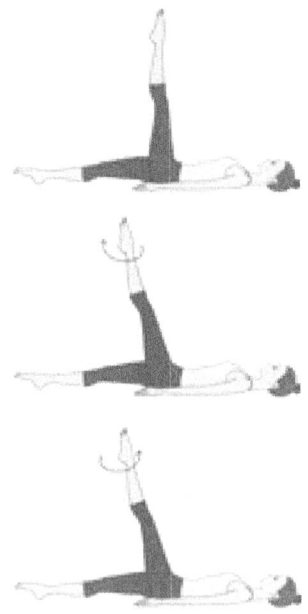

Leg circles are a Pilates exercise involving the circular movement of the legs, usually performed while lying on your back.

Benefits:

- Muscle strengthening. Leg circle exercises involve the abdominal, leg, buttock and hip muscles, contributing to their strengthening.
- Enhanced flexibility. Practicing this movement can contribute to improved flexibility in the hip joints and legs.
- Core Stability. Because it requires core control to maintain stability while performing leg circles, leg circles can help improve core strength and stability.
- Coordination development. Performing leg circles requires coordination between the leg and core muscles, thus helping to develop overall coordination of the body.
- Low Impact. It's a low-impact exercise, so it's relatively safe for many people, including those who may have joint or bone problems.

Execution:

1. Lie on your back with your arms along your body, palms on the ground and legs extended. One leg remains extended on the mat with the hammertoe (the heel on the ground and the toes pointing towards the ceiling), while the other leg is raised towards the ceiling with the toe extended.

2. With your leg raised, begin drawing small circles in the air with your toe. You can imagine drawing imaginary circles on the ceiling. Be sure to keep the rest of your body stable and still during this movement, focusing on engaging your hip and core muscles.
3. Inhaling, begin drawing the circle with your raised leg, slowly moving it outward and downward. Continue to inhale as you bring your leg into the first half of the circle. As you begin the second half of the circle, he begins to exhale slowly. Continue exhaling as you bring your leg up and inward, completing the circle.
4. Perform 5 complete circles in one direction, keeping the movement controlled and flowing. After that, reverse the direction of movement and perform 5 more complete circles in the opposite direction.
5. Repeat the same steps with the other leg, keeping the other side of your body stable and involved throughout the exercise.

Exercises to relieve stress and anxiety

Many people build up muscle tension due to chronic stress and anxiety. Somatic exercises include progressive muscle relaxation techniques, which involve consciously relaxing various muscle groups one at a time. This helps reduce physical tension and promotes a feeling of calm and relaxation.

Mindful movement is another pillar of somatic exercises to combat stress and anxiety. This type of movement involves conscious attention to the sensations and flow of movement, helping to reduce mental agitation and restore emotional balance.

Child Pose

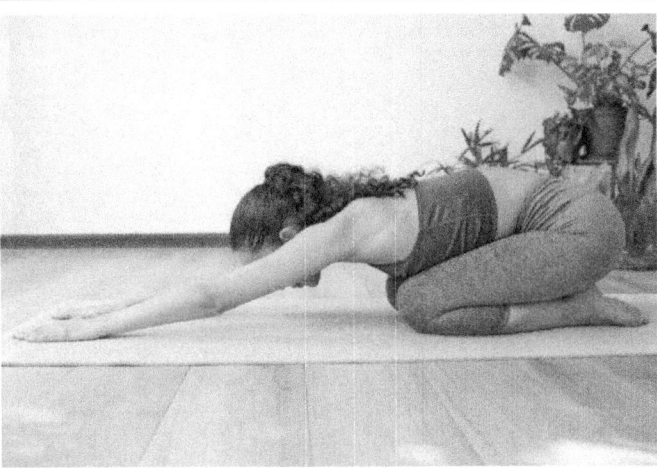

It is a somatic exercise thanks to which you can completely relax in a very short time; therefore, it is very useful for eliminating accumulated stress and fatigue.

This position is performed by both beginners and experts, not only because it allows a break between two challenging sequences, but also because it gives the practitioner countless benefits.

Benefits:

- Regular practice of Child's Pose allows the front of the torso to relax completely over the thighs, causing gentle compression of the front of the rib cage and abdominal. This action allows a delicate and healthy opening of the entire back part of the chest.
- When performing Balasana the forehead is placed on the ground and this places a slight pressure on the sixth Chakra, Anja, the center of intuition and creative imagination. The connection energy that develops allows you to turn your inner gaze towards your imagination, intuition and concentration.
- Precisely because of its crouched position, Balasana allows you to explore the healing power of breathing. In child pose you can direct your breath towards the back of the body, performing a beneficial internal massage on organs such as the kidneys and adrenal glands. Practiced in the evening it promotes sleep.

Execution:

1. Begin by positioning your knees on the ground and resting your pelvis on top of them. Your hands should be on the mat, shoulder-width apart, with your palms aligned with your hands. The big toes should be together.
2. At this point shift the weight of your hips back and comes to sit with your buttocks on your heels.
3. The arms can be placed in two positions either along the body, and in this case the palms are facing upwards, or you leave them stretched above the head, while in this case they are facing the ground.
4. The knees can be together or spread the same width as the mat.
5. At this point, let go of your entire torso and let your forehead touch the ground. If you can't touch, reach as far as you can and breathe deeply.
6. Try to focus on the back of your body and let any tension in your shoulders, back, neck and arms slowly disappear.
7. Now close your eyes, relax completely and hold Child's Pose as long as you need. Usually, it lasts two to five minutes, the time needed to relax.
8. To return to the starting position, push with your hands on the ground and straighten your torso, bringing it above your ankles.

Legs to the wall

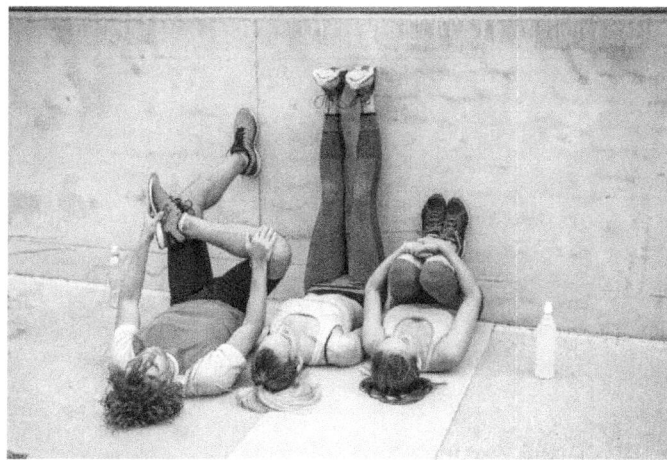

Viparita Karani, or legs to the wall, is a yoga position that involves elevating the legs in a supine position, often with the legs resting against a wall.

Benefits:

- The position of the legs against the wall promotes venous return, helping blood flow from the lower extremities to the heart. This can help improve blood circulation.
- By relieving tension and improving circulation, this pose can reduce swelling in the legs and feet.
- It can stimulate the digestive system, aiding in digestion and relieving any gastrointestinal disorders.

- The basic form of the position, with the legs resting against the wall, is known for its relaxing effect. This practice can aid in reducing anxiety and stress levels, fostering a general sense of calmness.
- By relieving pressure in the head and neck area, this pose can help relieve tension headaches.
- Thanks to its calming and relaxing effect, Viparita Karani can be useful in promoting sleep and combating insomnia.

Execution:

1. Lie your body on the mat, positioning yourself on your back with your stomach facing upwards.
2. Make sure you rest your back and buttocks well on the mat, maintaining a comfortable and aligned posture.
3. Start breathing consciously to increase concentration. Inhale and exhale slowly, synchronizing your breathing with your movements.
4. Gradually raise your legs straight up, utilizing your hands to support your lower back during this movement.
5. Place your palms just above your buttocks to support your body. Maintain your elbows flexed at approximately a 90-degree angle.
6. Gradually lower yourself to the floor, arching your back in a controlled manner. Ensure that your lower back is nearly parallel to the floor throughout this motion.

Box Breathing

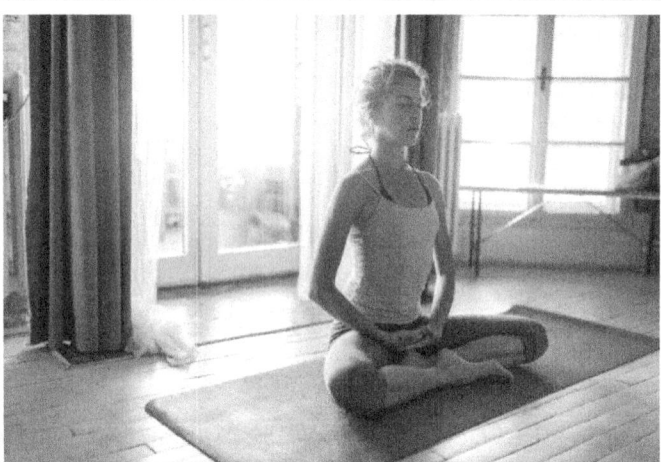

This technique is also called square breathing because each part of the breathing has the same timing as the others.

Benefits:

- This type of breathing helps anyone improve the management of their physical and mental resources. What it does, essentially, is balance the influence of the parasympathetic nervous system, which is calming and reduces the heart rate, with the sympathetic nervous system which is the typical one of the fight and flight response, which therefore, obviously, creates more tension. So, we can say that square breathing in its simplicity is very

useful for better dealing with any situation that requires an optimal balance between concentration and calm, between energy and control.
- Square breathing promotes mental focus through awareness of breathing and regulation of breathing rhythms. This can help improve concentration and attention.
- Regular practice of square breathing is associated with improved emotional control. Engaging in this practice can assist you in confronting stressful situations with enhanced mental clarity and emotional stability.
- Square breathing can increase brain oxygenation, providing more oxygen to brain cells. This can contribute to an increase in mental energy and vitality.
- Regular practice can help reduce levels of the stress hormone cortisol, promoting a more balanced physiological response to stressful situations.
- The practice of square breathing can be useful in promoting relaxation and preparing the body for restful sleep, thus contributing to improving the quality of sleep.

Execution:

The square breathing technique, composed of the four phases of inhalation, pause, exhalation and pause, is a practice that promotes conscious control of the breath.

1. Inhalation (Inhale). During inhalation, the body receives oxygen, essential nourishment for the optimal functioning of cells. Controlled inhalation helps increase the amount of oxygen reaching the blood, promoting vitality and energy.
2. Pause after Inhalation (Hold). The pause after inhaling allows the body to retain the freshly inhaled oxygen. This phase can promote the more effective distribution of oxygen in the circulatory system, improving the efficiency of the respiratory process.
3. Exhalation (Exhale). During exhalation, the body eliminates carbon dioxide, a byproduct of metabolism. Conscious exhaling can aid in relaxing the nervous system, alleviating tension, and fostering a state of calmness.
4. Pause after Exhalation (Hold). The pause after exhalation allows the body to remain in a state of temporary pulmonary vacuum. This stage can contribute to strengthening the diaphragm and enhancing overall lung capacity.
5. Repeat the exercise multiple times until you achieve a state of calmness and relaxation. Initially you can do 2 to 5 minutes of breathing.

Relaxing circle exercise

Relaxing circle exercise, or similar techniques involving visualization and awareness, can offer various mental and physical health benefits.

Benefits:

- The relaxing circle exercise is designed to calm the mind and reduce stress. Consistent practice can assist in decreasing levels of cortisol, the stress hormone, in the body.
- The mental and physical relaxation induced by this exercise can promote more restful sleep. Decreasing stress and calming the mind can enhance the quality of your sleep.
- Focused attention on the breath and visualization of the circle can increase awareness of the present moment. This type of awareness can lead to greater mental clarity and ability to deal with daily challenges.
- Regular practice can train your mind to focus on a single point, improving your concentration and ability to handle distractions.
- The relaxation hoop exercise can help relax muscles, reducing tension and muscle pain associated with stress.
- Reducing stress and increasing mindfulness can help manage anxiety symptoms. Constant practice can provide useful tools for dealing with anxious situations.

Execution:

1. Stand with your feet parallel and your hands alongside your body.
2. Ensure that you are in a comfortable and relaxed position.
3. Slowly bend your torso towards the left side, keeping your feet well anchored to the ground and your legs completely straight.
4. You can look towards the left side for more extension and elongation.
5. Slowly move your hands and torso in front of you, creating a semicircular motion.
6. Imagine drawing an imaginary circle with your hands as you move your torso.
7. Continue this movement until you reach the right side.
8. Upon reaching the right side, start the movement in the opposite direction.
9. Slowly move your hands and torso to the left side, following the semicircular path.
10. Coordinate the movement with deep breathing. For example, you might inhale as you extend your arms above your head and exhale as you bend to the side.
11. Maintain a slow, controlled pace to promote relaxation. Focus on the sensation of the movement and be aware of your muscles stretching and contracting.
12. After performing the desired number of repetitions, return to the standing position with your hands along your body.

Tree Pose

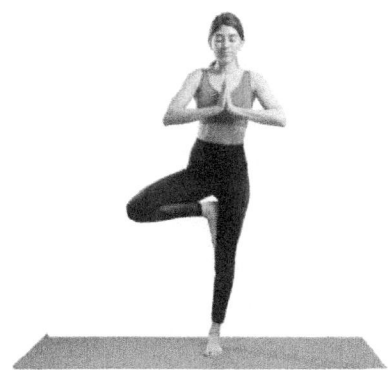

The Tree pose, known as Vrksasana in Sanskrit, is a fundamental yoga posture designed to enhance balance, stability, and concentration.

Benefits:

- Tree pose helps tone the front muscles of the thighs, especially the quadriceps, and helps stabilize the ankles.
- This position promotes a complete stretch of the back, thighs, groins and chest, helping to improve flexibility and mobility.
- Regular practice of tree pose can help relieve sciatica symptoms by reducing pressure on the sciatica and improving posture.
- Helps improve foot health, reducing problems such as flat feet, by activating and strengthening the muscles of the feet and ankles.
- The tree is known to improve body balance, as it requires concentration and stability during its execution.
- It can help correct unbalanced posture, as it promotes proper body alignment.
- Practicing tree pose can lead to a feeling of harmony and relaxation, as it promotes mental concentration and physical relaxation.
- Like many other yoga practices, tree pose can help reduce stress and anxiety, promoting a calmer, more peaceful state of mind.

Execution:

1. Stand with your feet positioned hip-width apart.
2. Shift your body weight onto your left foot, keeping your foot firmly rooted on the ground.
3. Lift your right leg, bending it at the knee, and hold the knee with both hands.
4. Push your knee towards your hands to straighten your leg, maintaining balance.
5. Rotate your right leg outward from the hip joint and rest the ball of your foot on the inside of your left thigh. Position the heel of your lifted leg close to your groin, ensuring that the knee of the raised leg is facing outward.
6. Place your palms together in front of your body, at heart level.

7. Balance in this position for a few deep, even breaths, keeping your body stable and focusing your gaze on a fixed point to help maintain balance.
8. To come out of the position, slowly release the raised leg and return it to the ground, returning to the standing position with both feet on the ground.
9. Repeat the process on the opposite side, lifting your left leg and repeating steps 3 through 7.

The movement of the Flowing River

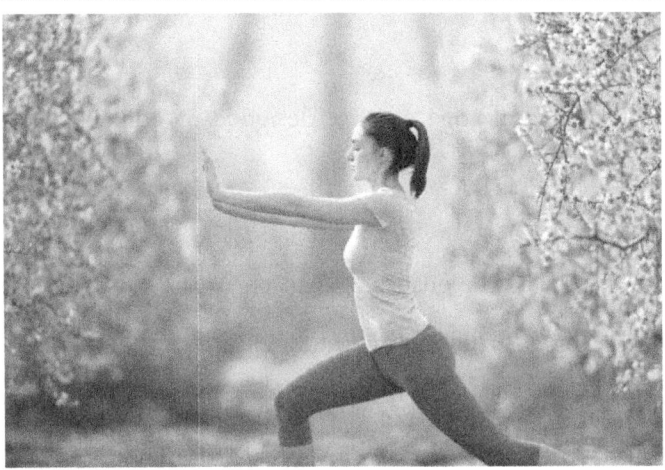

The flowing river movement, also known as "Floating Arms" or "Wave Hands Like Clouds," is a foundational exercise in Tai Chi that offers numerous health and wellness benefits.

Benefits:

- The movement of the flowing river involves fluid and harmonious movements of the arms, accompanied by deep and conscious breathing. This combination helps reduce stress, anxiety and mental tension, inducing a state of calm and relaxation.
- The circular motion of the arms in the flowing river helps improve the flexibility and mobility of the shoulder, elbow and wrist joints. This can be particularly beneficial for individuals experiencing stiffness or tension in their joints.
- Although Tai Chi is generally considered a low-intensity exercise, the flowing river movement still involves activating and toning the muscles of the arms, shoulders and core. This can help improve muscle strength and endurance over time.
- Since the motion of the flowing river requires precise coordination of arm movements and breathing, it can help improve hand-eye coordination and balance. This aspect is particularly important for older adults or individuals seeking to enhance stability and body awareness.

- The constant movement of the arms in the flowing river helps stimulate blood circulation throughout the body. This can help improve blood flow to the extremities and increase tissue oxygenation, promoting cardiovascular and overall health.
- Practicing the flowing river movement requires mental focus and awareness of the present moment. This can help promote mental calm, concentration and mental clarity, improving your ability to manage stress and distractions.

Execution:

1. Begin by standing with your feet slightly apart, aligned with your hips. Relax your arms at your sides, keeping them slightly bent at the elbows.
2. Inhaling slowly, begin to lift your arms in front of you, bringing them up and over your head. Your hands should remain together or slightly apart, with palms facing the ceiling. Continue to raise your arms until they are fully extended above your head, keeping your shoulders relaxed.
3. As you exhale, begin to rotate your arms down and away from your body in a circular motion. Your hands should move together, keeping your fingers slightly open and your palms facing the floor. Continue the circular motion until your arms come back to the starting position at your sides.
4. Repeat the movement smoothly and continuously, synchronizing the movement with your breathing. Inhaling as you lift your arms straight up and exhaling as you move your arms downward and sideways in a circular motion from your body.
5. Focus your attention on the flow of the circular motion of your arms, imagining yourself as a gently flowing river. Feel the fluidity and lightness of movement as you move through the space. Additionally, maintain deep, regular breathing, synchronizing each movement with your inhalation and exhalation.
6. As you perform the movement, maintain a focused mental awareness of the present moment. Let go of any tension or worry and allow your mind to be calm and present in movement and breathing.
7. You can repeat the movement of the flowing river for several minutes, focusing on the sensation of relaxation and fluidity.

The 5-4-3-2-1 Grounding Technique

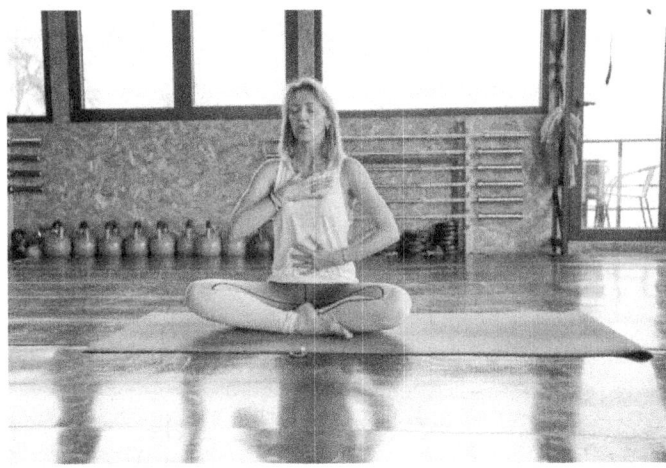

The 5-4-3-2-1 grounding technique is a self-help practice used to calm anxiety and reconnect with the present moment. It is based on the idea of using the senses to focus attention on immediate physical sensations, thus reducing stress and anxiety.

Benefits:

- By focusing on your senses and physical sensations in the present moment, you can interrupt the flow of anxious thoughts and worries, thus reducing anxiety.
- The practice of 5-4-3-2-1 grounding assists in heightening your awareness of your senses and your environment. This can lead to greater awareness of yourself and your experiences.
- Focusing attention on the senses can act as a positive distraction from worries and negative moods. This can help you break negative thought cycles.
- Regular grounding practice can help you develop emotional self-regulation skills, allowing you to better manage stress. anxiety and intense emotions.

Execution:

1. 5, things you see. Begin by observing five objects in your vicinity. The objects can vary in size and type. It doesn't matter what they are, big or small. Concentrate on the details of each object, observing its color, shape and texture. Make a conscious effort to concentrate your attention on these objects.
2. 4, things you touch. Now, focus your attention on four things you can physically touch. It could be the texture of your dress, the surface of a table, or anything else. Focus on physical sensations and be aware of how they feel to the touch.
3. 3, things you feel. Take note of three sounds around you. They could be ambient sounds, such as traffic noise, the rustle of the wind or someone's voice. Be mindful of the sounds present in your surroundings at that particular moment.
4. 2, things you smell. Pay attention to two odors in the environment. It could be the fragrance of a flower, the aroma of freshly brewed coffee, or any other scent you detect. Breathe deeply and focus on these smells.

5. 1, things you savor. Finally, focus your attention on the taste in your mouth. It could be the taste of a meal you just ate, the taste of toothpaste, or any other taste present.
6. Mentally repeat each step, allowing yourself to fully explore and notice the details of your surroundings. This technique aids in interrupting the flow of anxious thoughts, guiding you back to the present moment through your senses.

Butterfly hug

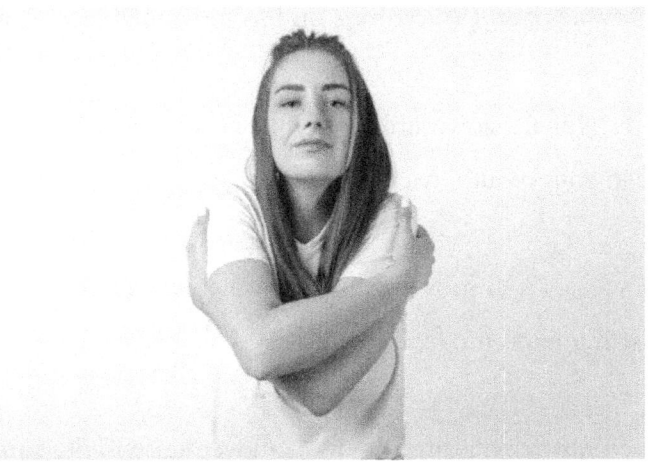

Butterfly hug is a very simple technique to calm yourself down when you feel overwhelmed by anxiety. The butterfly hug works by touching both sides of the chest and is designed to help the nervous system calm down during times of increased stress or anxiety.

The Butterfly Hug technique was initially developed for a therapeutic approach called Eye Movement Desensitization and Reprocessing (EMDR), utilized to assist individuals in processing painful or traumatic memories. This technique operates through bilateral stimulation, wherein a stimulus is administered alternately to both sides of the body.

Benefits:

- The butterfly hug can help relax your shoulder and neck muscles, reducing built-up tension. This can aid in reducing stress and anxiety, as relaxed muscles are frequently linked with a heightened sense of calm.
- This technique can increase body awareness, helping people connect with the physical sensations of their body. This can be especially helpful for those who tend to ignore physical sensations or hold emotional tension in the body.
- The butterfly hug can stimulate the production of endorphins, chemicals in the brain associated with feelings of well-being and happiness.

Execution:

1. Find a quiet place where you can sit or stand comfortably. Position your hands so your thumbs meet, then place them gently on your sternum, with your hands resting on your chest and your fingertips lightly touching your collarbones. Ensure that you are in a relaxed position with a comfortable posture.
2. Once your hands are positioned correctly, take a moment to feel the contact of your hands with your body. The light pressure on the sternum and the fingertips touching the collarbones can feel like a light and reassuring hug.
3. Start a gentle, rhythmic movement with your hands, mimicking the fluttering of a butterfly's wings. Alternate with gently tapping your chest, maintaining a comfortable pace. Concentrate on this movement, trying to be aware of each touch and the rhythm you are creating.
4. While moving your hands, synchronize deep breaths. Inhale slowly through your nose, feeling your chest expand as air fills your lungs. Exhale gradually through your mouth, releasing any tension or worries. This will help intensify the relaxing effect of the exercise.
5. Find a pace that works for you. Some people may prefer a faster movement, while others may find benefit in a slower, calming pace. Experiment with and adjust the hand movement and speed to suit your individual needs and preferences.
6. If you are in an environment where you don't feel comfortable performing this movement visibly, you can alternate tapping on the outside of your knees. This movement is more subtle but can still provide a similar feeling of comfort and relaxation.

Fish Pose

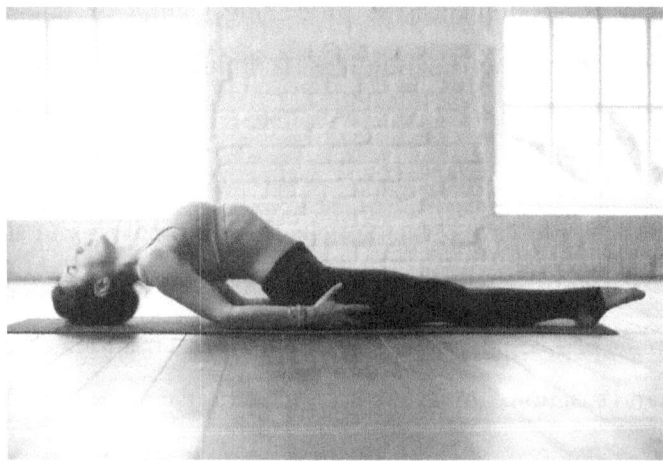

Fish pose, or Matsyasana in yoga, is a pose that can be used to relax and open the chest area, improve breathing, and relieve discomfort associated with stress and anxiety.

Benefits:

- The fish pose entails a profound opening of the chest, which can enhance breathing capacity. Engaging in deep, mindful breathing can aid in alleviating tension and anxiety, fostering a sense of calmness.
- Practicing Matsyasana requires awareness and attention to the body. This increase in body awareness can help focus the mind on the present moment, thus reducing anxiety related to future thoughts or worries.

Execution:

1. Lie on the mat with your back straight and your legs extended in front of you and your hands under your buttocks with palms facing down, shoulders and neck relaxed. This step is not to be underestimated, it is very important to become aware of the upper and lower parts of the body at the same time.
2. Bring your shoulders back and down and pushing your forearms and hands onto the floor. Lift your chest and head, arch your spine slightly, make sure your elbows are perpendicular to your forearms. Keep your head aligned straight and direct your gaze forward. The legs and feet stretch a lot, which helps the spine arch more.
3. Arch your spine as much as possible, open your chest more by pushing from your elbows, if necessary, slide them forward a little more, and bring the top of your head to the floor.
4. Continue stretching your legs and feet. Try not to carry too much weight just on your head but distribute it throughout your body so as not to put too much strain on your neck. Remain in this position for a while, continuing to breathe regularly.

Corpse Pose

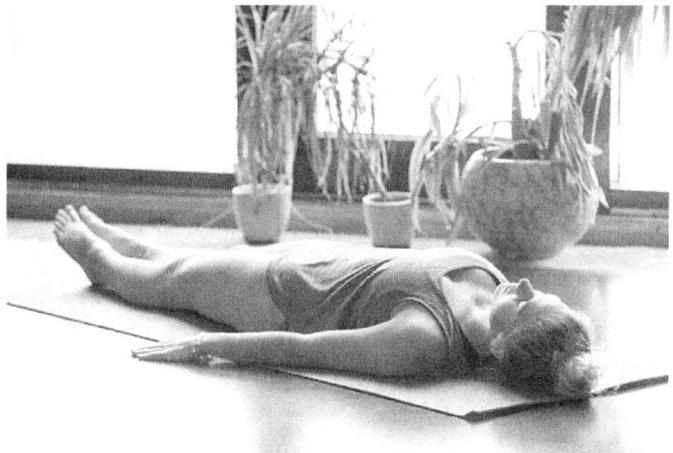

Savasana is also called corpse pose or relaxation pose and is a basic pose in Hatha Yoga.

Benefits:

- The most important benefit of Savasana, as the name of relaxation position itself suggests, is precisely that of creating physical and mental relaxation. Savasana is designed to promote deep relaxation. Remaining in this position allows the body to release muscle tension and activate the parasympathetic nervous system, thus reducing stress and anxiety.

- During Savasana, your attention is turned inward, encouraging awareness of your body, breathing and mental state. This can help you develop greater body awareness, an important asset in managing anxiety.
- Savasana promotes slow, deep breathing. Focusing on mindful breathing helps regulate the nervous system, reducing the heart rate and muscle tension associated with anxiety.

Executions:

1. First, lie down on the mat gently.
2. Now bend your knees and bring them to your chest. You will notice how this simple movement causes the lumbar area to relax further. At this point, slowly extend one leg at a time, bringing them both back to the ground so that they are slightly apart.
3. Relax both legs, allowing your toes to rotate slightly outward. Make sure they are open and rotated equally. If they aren't, adjust as best you can to make sure they are.
4. Now focus on the shoulder area. It is important that they are open and relaxed. To help you open, you can raise your arms to a position perpendicular to the floor. This simple gesture will help you open your shoulder blades and, therefore, this entire area. Now, keeping your shoulders still, gently bring your arms to the ground, positioning them at the sides of your body at the same distance. At this point let them relax and open outwards. Use your mind and breath to help them relax further.
5. Now bring your attention to your neck. The latter should be erect so that the two ears are the same distance from each shoulder. Try to stretch your entire neck so that it is both stretched and relaxed.
6. Finally, you need to focus on the head. It is important that you are able to relax all your facial muscles and also your sense organs. Bring your attention first to the tongue, relaxing it, and then to the eyes, turning your gaze inward.
7. Let the breath come in and out naturally, without forcing it in any way.
8. Leave the body totally abandoned on the ground. Feel the weight of your head and allow it to relax further with each breath, becoming heavier and more relaxed.
9. Remain in this position for a minimum of 10 minutes. A general rule is that you should hold Savasana for 5 minutes every 30 minutes of practice.
10. To exit the corpse position, begin to move your feet, hands and neck slightly. Now, gently rotate your entire body to the right and hold this position for a few breaths. Then, utilizing primarily your left hand, gradually stand up and return to a seated position.

Mountain Pose

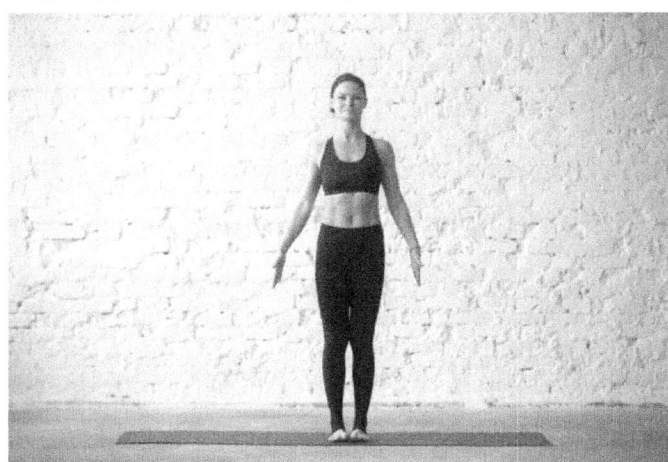

Mountain pose is a yoga practice that involves standing upright, with feet firmly rooted to the ground, shoulders extended, chest raised, and arms at your sides or raised above your head. It is one of the basic positions in yoga and is named so because it emulates the stability and solidity of the mountains.

Benefits:

- Mountain pose helps realign the spine, improving posture and reducing the risk of muscle tension and pain.
- This pose actively involves the muscles of the legs, core, and arms, aiding in strengthening and toning the body.
- The mountain pose encourages deep and mindful breathing, which can help to calm the mind and alleviate stress.
- Holding mountain pose requires concentration and presence of mind, which can help improve concentration and focus on daily life.
- Standing still in this position helps improve balance and physical stability, useful for preventing falls and improving performance in other sporting activities.

Execution:

1. Start standing, with your feet together or slightly hip-width apart. Distribute your weight evenly across both feet and sense the roots of your soles grounding into the ground.
2. Lengthen the spine. Imagine stretching your head toward the ceiling as you align your shoulders with your hips. Relax your shoulders and maintain a lifted chest.
3. Relax your arms at your sides or bring your hands together behind your back, with fingers interlocked, if that feels more comfortable.
4. Focus your gaze in front of you, on a fixed point, keeping your gaze soft and relaxed.
5. Make sure your knees are slightly bent, without locking them completely. Maintain the alignment of your knees with your ankles and hips.

6. Engage your abdominal and core muscles but avoid overly tensing. Strive to maintain a balance between strength and relaxation.
7. Inhale deeply and slowly through your nose, allowing your lungs to fill completely. Exhale slowly through your nose or mouth, releasing any tension in your body.
8. Hold Mountain Pose for at least 30 seconds or more, breathing consciously and maintaining good posture.
9. To come out of the pose, slowly release your arms to your sides and return to the upright standing position.

Exercises for flexibility and stretch

Flexibility is a fundamental element of physical health and well-being, helping to improve posture, prevent muscle injuries and improve athletic performance. Somatic exercises offer a dynamic approach to stretching that goes beyond simply lengthening muscles. Effective stretching also requires relaxing the muscles involved in the movement. Somatic exercises include progressive muscle relaxation techniques and consciously relaxing the muscles while stretching, helping to improve flexibility and reduce feelings of tension.

Feldenkrais Thoracic rotation

Feldenkrais thoracic rotation involves conscious and gentle movements of the upper body, particularly the thoracic or chest region. Through targeted exercises and guided movement sequences, we aim to improve flexibility, coordination and awareness of rotation in the thoracic area. This can be particularly useful for people who have tension or limitations in chest movements, which can arise from various causes such as stress, poor posture or muscle problems.

Benefits:

- It helps people become more aware of their movements and sensations in the chest area.
- The goal is to increase the flexibility and mobility of the thoracic spine to promote more fluid and natural movements.
- The practice aims to reduce muscle tension and relieve any pain or stiffness in the thoracic region.
- It helps improve overall posture and coordination in upper trunk movements.

Execution:

1. Start with a slow, controlled rotation of your head to the right. Ensure not to force the movement and pay close attention to the sensations in your neck and shoulders as you rotate.
2. Fixate on a specific point on the wall, perhaps at eye level. Look at details like the shape, color, or any distinguishing features of that spot.
3. Repeat the movement, rotating your head to the left as far as you comfortably can. Once again, choose a point on the wall to focus on. Memorize both points in your mind for later comparison.
4. Place your arms crossed over your chest comfortably. Keep your head aligned with your body, avoiding any rotation of your head during this step.
5. Rotate your body to the right, focusing on the sensation of lengthening and opening along your chest. You can fix your gaze on a landmark to maintain direction awareness.
6. Next, rotate your body to the left. Once again, choose a point on the wall as a reference. Memorizes the reference points chosen during both rotations.

7. Return to the starting position by crossing your arms over your chest. Now, rotate your head backwards, either to the left or to the right. Assess if you notice an improvement in your range of motion compared to the initial step.

8. Be aware of any sensations of increased flexibility or reduced tension in the neck and shoulder regions. Mentally compare the reference points chosen during head rotation with those memorized in step 1 to evaluate any improvements in your rotation ability.

The Saw

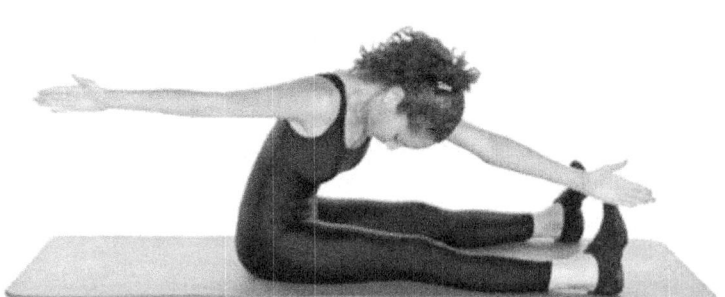

The Saw is a Pilates exercise designed to improve spinal flexibility, strengthen core muscles and increase body awareness. This exercise involves torso rotation and lateral flexion, working different parts of the body simultaneously.

Benefits:

- The exercise involves spinal rotation and lateral flexion, helping to improve spinal flexibility and thoracic mobility.
- The Saw requires activation of the abdominal and core muscles to maintain control during rotation and lateral bending. This exercise aids in developing strength and stability in the core region of the body.
- The exercise also engages the leg adductors and lateral muscles, contributing to muscle lengthening and improving flexibility in the hip area.
- Attention to correct posture during execution can contribute to the general improvement of posture, as you work on awareness of the position of the torso and spine.

Execution:

1. Sit on the floor with your legs apart, keeping your spine lengthened. Open your arms to the side with your shoulders soft and shoulder blades close together. This position provides a stable base for performing subsequent exercises.

2. Begin by inhaling deeply and extending your spine upward, preparing for the movement. Bring attention to your posture and maintaining a long position.
3. Exhale as you begin to twist your torso to the right. The arms move in tandem with the torso, accentuating the engagement of the entire upper body. Continue twisting until your head is aligned with your right foot. Hold the position with control.
4. Again, inhale while extending your spine, preparing for the second movement. Keep your posture long and focus on pelvic stability.
5. Exhale keeping your buttocks on the ground and flex your torso forward. Focus on bending from your lower back and continue lowering yourself, trying to bring your chest closer to her thigh. Keep your spine extended without contracting your shoulders.
6. Extend your left hand towards your right foot while simultaneously extending your right arm back. This movement adds a component of lateral bending and twisting, further engaging the upper body muscles.
7. Repeat the entire exercise 10 times on both sides, alternating the use of your arms.
8. Maintain a steady, fluid pace, avoiding long pauses between repetitions to maintain the intensity of the exercise.
9. Pay particular attention to your breathing, synchronizing it with your movements. Inhalation should be associated with extension, while exhalation is associated with twisting and forward bending.
10. Be careful to maintain good posture and adapt to your individual limitations of movement, avoiding excessive tension or sudden movements.

Mermaid

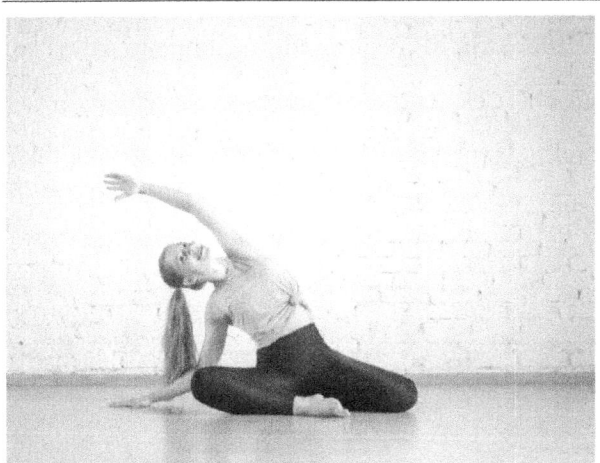

The Mermaid exercise is a Pilates movement that combines lateral bending and rotation of the torso to improve flexibility and strength in the upper body. This exercise can be executed either on a Pilates mat or using a specially designed Pilates chair.

Benefits:

- The exercise involves significant lateral flexion of the torso, helping to improve the flexibility of the spine in the lateral direction.
- During the movement, the core muscles, especially the obliques, are activated to stabilize the spine and support lateral movement.
- The exercise also engages the adductors, the inner thigh muscles, when changing the position of the legs.
- The rotation movement of the torso favors the involvement of the chest muscles, contributing to the mobility of the upper back.

Execution:
1. Sit on the floor on your left side with your legs bent and drawn towards the right side of your body.
2. The right-hand rests on the right ankle, creating support to maintain the position.
3. Maintain an upright posture with an elongated spine and shoulders kept relaxed.
4. Flex your torso in the direction of your legs (i.e. to the right). Activate the muscles in the waist area on the right side, imagining that you are holding an object between your ribs and your right hip.
5. Continue to exhale as you move your torso down and to the right, trying to bring your chest closer to your knees. This motion entails lateral flexion of the spine.
6. Keep your left arm straight overhead to accentuate lateral flexion and maintain the lengthening of the left side of your body.
7. Gradually return to the starting position, lengthening your torso and raising your right arm straight up. Keep your right-side muscles contracting to support the movement.
8. Bring your right forearm to the ground, raising your torso.
9. Flex your torso in the opposite direction, lowering your left forearm to the ground. Continue to exhale as you move your torso down and to the left, trying to bring your chest closer to your knees.
10. Keep your right arm straight overhead to accentuate lateral flexion and maintain the lengthening of the right side of your body.

Forward Fold

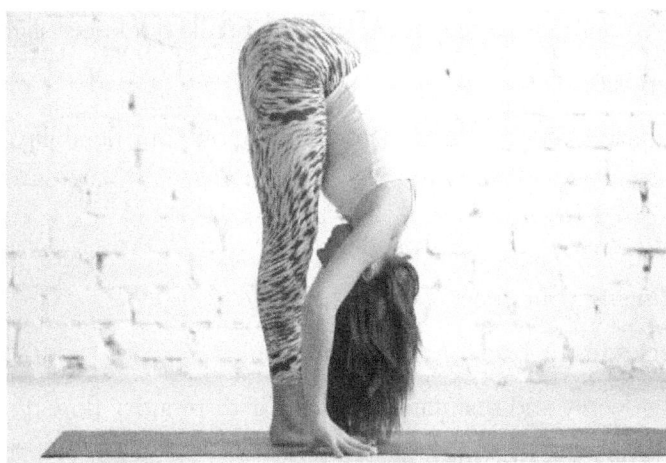

Forward Fold or forward bend is an important position in yoga, also known as Uttanasana. This position offers numerous benefits for the body and mind and is often included in yoga sequences to improve flexibility, lengthen the leg and back muscles, and bring positive effects to the spine.

Benefits:

- Uttanasana involves a deep stretch of the back muscles of the legs, including the calves, hamstrings, and lower back muscles.
- This position encourages the extension of the spine, fostering flexibility and mobility in this region.
- Uttanasana is effective in relaxing and stretching the muscles of the shoulders, back and legs, reducing muscle tension.
- The position lightly compresses the abdomen, stimulating the internal organs, improving digestion and promoting a healthy digestive system.
- The soothing nature of Uttanasana aids in calming the mind, alleviating stress and anxiety. Leaning forward is often associated with the release of mental tension.
- The posture encourages enhanced blood circulation to the brain, facilitating improved concentration and mental clarity.
- Depending on the variation of Uttanasana, such as reaching the hands behind the back, a lengthening and opening of the shoulders can be achieved.

Execution:

1. Begin by standing with your feet positioned hip-width apart.
2. Maintain an upright posture with relaxed shoulders and a long spine.
3. Inhaling deeply, bring your attention to your breathing and posture.
4. Prepare your body for forward movement by lightly activating your core muscles.
5. As you exhale, begin to bend your torso forward from the waist, bringing your chest towards your thighs.

6. Try to keep your legs straight, but if flexibility limits your ability to keep them straight, bend your knees slightly. The goal is to attain a comfortable and sustainable position.
7. Place your hands on your thighs, on the floor, or grasp opposite forearms depending on your flexibility and comfort.
8. Let your head and neck be relaxed, avoiding holding tension in your shoulders.
9. Try to lengthen your back as you bend forward, bringing your chest towards your legs.
10. Gradually relax into the position, allowing the muscles in the back of your legs to lengthen.
11. Hold the position for at least 20 seconds, breathing deeply and maintaining a regular respiratory flow. Focus on the sensation of stretching and the progressive relaxation of your muscles.
12. Inhale slowly as you start to rise back to a standing position. Utilize your abdominal muscles to gradually lift your torso upward. Maintain control of the movement to avoid sudden returns to a standing position.

Eagle Pose

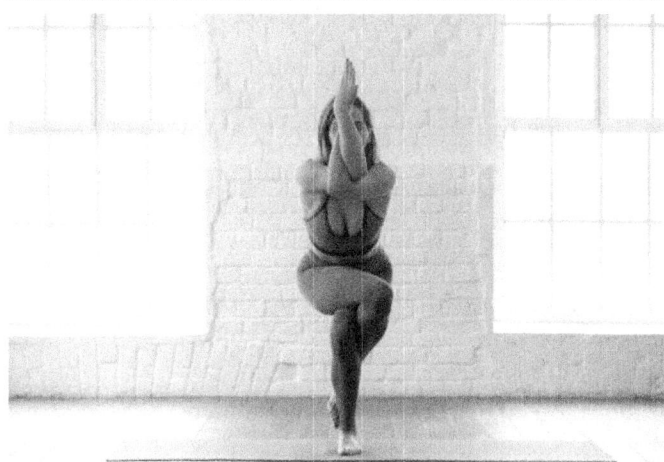

Eagle pose, or "Garudasana" in Sanskrit, is a yoga pose that involves twisting the arms and legs, with the arms crossed in front of the body and the legs intertwined.

Benefits:

- The eagle pose requires good balance and concentration. Regular practice of this pose can aid in enhancing both physical and mental stability. Leg and arm braiding engages the leg and back muscles, helping to strengthen these areas of the body.
- The intertwining of the legs and arms can help stimulate blood circulation, promoting the flow of blood through the body.
- The act of crossing your arms in front of your body during this pose helps lengthen and open your shoulders and upper back, helping to improve flexibility in these areas.

- The act of rotating your neck slightly during eagle pose can help release built-up tension in the neck and shoulder region.

Execution:

1. Start standing. You have your feet close together, arms at your sides, and your weight evenly distributed on both feet.
2. Transfer your body weight onto your left foot and position your hands on your waist. Distribute your weight evenly across your left leg as you lift your right foot.
3. Bend your knees slightly while keeping your gaze fixed on a fixed point to help with balance.
4. Cross your right leg over your left, overlapping your thighs. Try to hook your feet around the ankle of the opposite leg.
5. Raise your arms in front of you, then cross your left arm under your right.
6. Bend your elbows and try to bring your palms together.
7. Remain in this position for 15-20 seconds. With each inhalation, try to lift your elbows slightly and move your arms away from your body.
8. Inhale and exhale as you release your arms and legs, returning to the starting position.
9. Change your body weight to your right leg, lift your left leg, cross it over your right and repeat the sequence.

Cow Pose

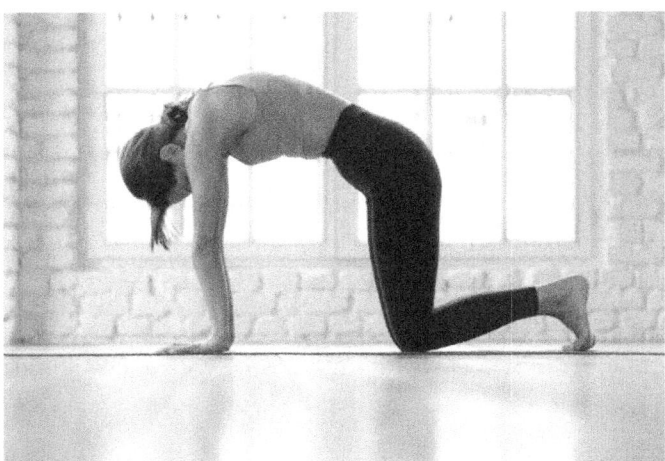

Bitilasana, also known as the cow pose, is a yoga exercise that offers several benefits for the body and mind.

Benefits:

- Bitilasana involves fluid movements of the spine, helping to increase flexibility and improve back mobility.
- Regular practice of Bitilasana can help improve body coordination and promote a more correct posture.
- During Bitilasana, the abdominal organs are activated and strengthened, contributing to better stability and support of the central region of the body.

- The exercise actively engages your core muscles, including your abdominal, obliques, and lower back muscles, helping to strengthen this important area of the body.
- The rhythmic movements of the spine during Bitilasana promote lengthening and greater flexibility of the spine.
- During execution, the arms, shoulders and wrists support the weight of the body, contributing to their strengthening and toning.
- The practice of Bitilasana, together with deep and conscious breathing, can help reduce stress, calm the mind and promote a sense of calm, thus helping to improve the quality of sleep.
- Thanks to the combination of fluid movements, conscious breathing and mental concentration, Bitilasana is effective in reducing stress and promoting a feeling of calm and mental well-being.

Execution:
1. Assume the position on the mat with your hands beneath your shoulders and your knees beneath your hips, creating an all-fours stance. Ensure that your wrists are aligned with your elbows and your knees are aligned with your hips.
2. Make sure your body is aligned correctly. Hands under shoulders and wrists under elbows, knees under hips. Maintain a flat back and ensure that your neck is aligned with your spine.
3. Inhale as you tilt your pelvis down, pushing your abdomen and chest slightly toward the floor. Lift your chin and look forward, slightly stretching your neck.
4. Continue to inhale as you lengthen your spine, allowing your back to arch downward slightly. You may experience a gentle stretch in the front of your body and a sensation of opening in your chest.
5. As you exhale, tilt your pelvis upwards and round your back, bringing your chin towards your chest. Contract your abs slightly as you lift the center of your chest toward the ceiling, creating a curve in your upper back.
6. Continue moving back and forth between these two positions, synchronizing the movement with your breathing: inhale as you lean forward and exhale as you tilt your pelvis upward.
7. You may choose to remain in each position for a few breaths, feeling the muscles of your back, shoulders, and abdominals stretch and strengthen.
8. After performing several repetitions, return to the neutral all-fours position and relax for a few breaths, observing the sensations in your body.

Spine Stretch Forward

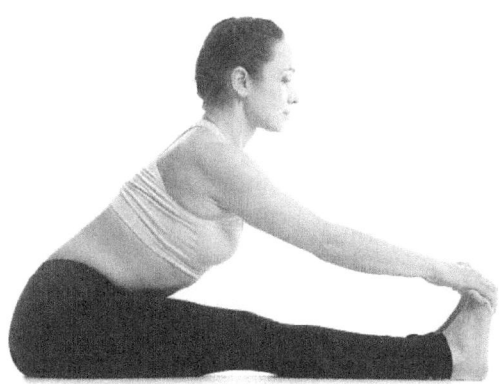

The spine stretch is an exercise that can help improve the flexibility of the spine and relieve any tension in the neck and shoulder areas.

Benefits:

- During the spine stretch, the movement involves a forward flexion of the spine, helping to extend and lengthen the vertebrae. This can be especially beneficial for those who spend a lot of time in a sitting position or have a posture that can cause spinal compression.
- Spine stretch can help relax the muscles in the neck and shoulder area, especially when the movement is performed in a controlled and conscious manner. This can be helpful in relieving tension built up in these areas.
- The forward bending movement during the spine stretch also involves the thoracic region of the spine. This can help improve the flexibility of this area, which is often limited in people who spend a lot of time in seated positions or with a forward posture.
- Integrating the spine stretch into your routine can help improve posture awareness and promote more correct alignment of the spine in everyday life.

Execution:

1. Position yourself on the floor with your legs spread apart, approximately shoulder-width apart. Alternatively, you can use a yoga mat for this exercise.
2. Ensure that your knees are slightly bent, permitting your pelvis to naturally tilt forward.
3. Extend your arms in front of you and grasp your wrists or toes. If you're unable to reach your feet, you can hold onto your ankles or legs, while maintaining a straight back.
4. As you inhale, lengthen your spine so your head stretches upward.
5. Exhaling, bend your torso forward from the pelvis, trying to bring your chest towards your knees.
6. Maintain a straight back throughout this initial phase of the movement.

7. Continue exhaling and flexing your spine gradually, allowing your head to move closer to the floor. Attempt to keep your shoulders relaxed and avoid unnecessary tension.
8. Reach maximum flexion, holding the position for a few deep breaths. Try to maintain spinal alignment.
9. At the end of the inhalation, rise back to a standing position while keeping your back straight.
10. Repeat the movement for several repetitions, maintaining a controlled and conscious rhythm. You can gradually intensify the movement as your flexibility improves over time.

Arm Swings

The arm swings exercise involves moving your arms back and forth in a swinging manner. It can be performed standing or seated, with the arms are swinging back and forth through a full range of shoulder motion.

Benefits:
- Arm swings are effective in warming up the muscles of the arms, shoulders and chest before more intense physical activity. This helps prepare the muscles for exertion and reduces the risk of injury.
- The dynamic movement of the arms promotes blood circulation in this area, helping to improve blood flow and supply oxygen to the muscles.
- Arm swings involve a full range of shoulder motion, helping to improve the mobility and flexibility of this area.
- During the movement of the arms backwards, the back muscles are activated, favoring the strengthening and involvement of the posterior muscles.
- The rocking motion can help reduce tension built up in the shoulders and neck, especially beneficial for those who spend a lot of time in sedentary or working positions. The lower back can also benefit from arm swings, as the movement involves rotation of the trunk, helping to relax the lower back.
- The exercise also engages the core muscles during trunk rotation, helping to strengthen the abdominal region.
- Arm swings can help improve coordination between arm and trunk movements.

Execution:
1. Stand with your knees slightly bent, keeping your feet shoulder-width apart.
2. Extend your arms horizontally towards the sides, keeping them parallel to the floor.
3. Cross your arms in front of you, bringing one above and one below, and then quickly bring them back to the starting position.
4. Maintain constant, fluid movement of your arms throughout the exercise.
5. Keep your abdominal muscles engaged to stabilize your core.
6. Keep your back straight, avoiding excessive leaning forward or backward.

7. Your torso should remain upright, with your gaze directed forward to maintain spinal alignment.
8. The knees are slightly bent to reduce strain on the joints.
9. Distribute your weight evenly between both feet.
10. Use the muscles in your arms and shoulders to push the movement of your arms back and forth.
11. Avoid sudden or excessively fast movements that could increase the risk of injury.
12. Breathe slowly and in a controlled manner throughout the movement.
13. Coordinate your breathing with the movement of your arms: for example, inhale when your arms cross in front and exhale when your arms return.
14. Keep your abs tight as you breathe to engage your core and support core stability.
15. Avoid raising your shoulders excessively during the movement. Keep your shoulders relaxed and drawn down to avoid unnecessary tension.
16. Try to bring your arms through their full range of motion, aiming for maximum opening and closing throughout the movement.
17. You can tailor the number of repetitions based on your fitness level and specific training objectives.

Single Leg Stretch

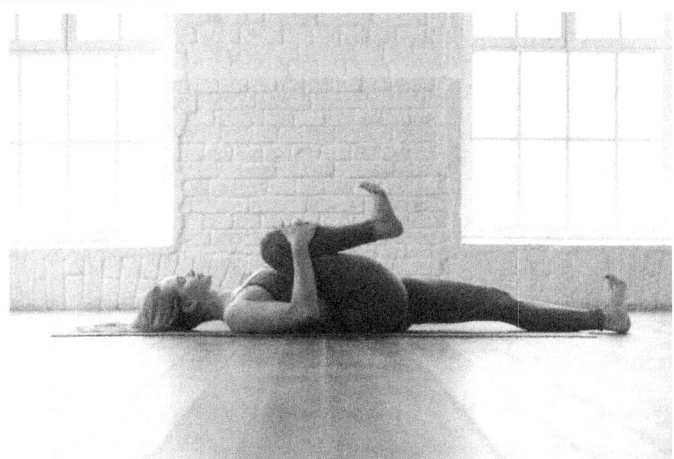

Single Leg Stretch is a Pilates exercise that engages the abdominal and leg muscles. Practicing this exercise can offer several benefits for the body.

Benefits:

- The single leg stretch is specifically designed to target abdominal strength. These muscles are essential for supporting the spine and maintaining correct posture.
- The extension and retraction of the legs involved in the single leg stretch require the use of the leg muscles, including the quadriceps and hamstrings. This can help improve leg strength and tone.

- When performing the single leg stretch, the spine is involved in flexion and extension movements. This can help improve spinal flexibility and reduce stiffness.
- The exercise requires precise coordination between the upper and lower limbs, as well as muscle control to avoid excessive movement. This can help improve the overall coordination of the body.
- The single leg stretch is an exercise that involves the core, including the abdominals, lower back and lateral muscles. Strengthening your core is essential to support your posture, improve balance and prevent any back problems.

Execution:
1. Lie on your back on an exercise mat, with your legs fully extended and your arms resting at your sides.
2. Keep your toes pulled down, your neck long and your head on the ground.
3. Inhaling, prepare for the movement by bringing your belly in, engaging your abdominal muscles and slowly lifting your shoulders off the floor.
4. At the same time, he lifts his left leg off the floor, bringing his knee towards his chest. Keep the other leg fully extended.
5. Exhale, keeping his stomach in, and grips your left knee with both hands. Keep your head, neck, and shoulders lifted off the floor.
6. Inhale deeply while maintaining the position, focusing on controlled breathing.
7. As you exhale, bring your bent left knee towards your chest while simultaneously extending your right leg upward.
8. Keep your pelvis stable and ensure your lower back remains flat against the floor.
9. Avoid pulling your head with your hands; instead, engage your abdominal muscles to lift your upper body.
10. Focus attention on the quality of movement, maintaining fluidity and control.
11. Inhale as you return to the starting position, maintaining control of the abdominal contraction.
12. Repeat the entire movement with the other leg, raising your right leg, bringing your right knee to your chest, and alternating legs.
13. For beginners, perform the exercise for 5 repetitions with each leg.
14. For advanced levels, gradually increase the number of repetitions up to 10 with each leg.

Raised arm Pose

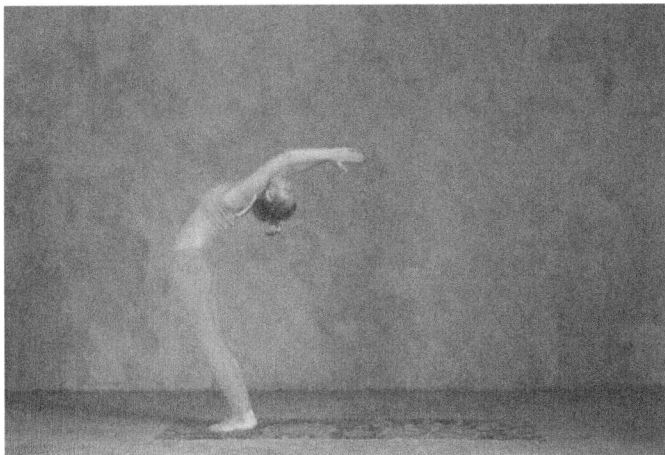

Hasta Uttanasana, or the Standing Bend or Raised Arm Pose, is a yoga pose that offers a variety of physical and mental benefits.

Benefits:

- During Hasta Uttanasana, the forward-leaning motion helps relax and stimulate the back muscles, improving the flexibility of the spine and increasing blood circulation in the area.
- The forward lean during Hasta Uttanasana creates a deep stretch of the abdominal and viscera, promoting blood flow to the internal organs and improving digestive health.
- By raising your arms above your head and leaning forward, Hasta Uttanasana opens your chest, improving lung capacity and promoting deeper, more effective breathing.
- The pose stimulates the spinal cord and the sympathetic nervous system, aiding in body relaxation and stress reduction.
- By regularly performing Hasta Uttanasana, you can help keep your back aligned and healthy, preventing or reducing the risk of problems with your spine and surrounding muscles.
- The forward lean helps to relax and stretch the muscles of the back and shoulders, helping to correct any curvature or tension and promoting a more upright and balanced posture.

Execution:

1. Start standing, with your feet parallel and slightly apart, aligned with your hips. Keep your arms at your sides, with shoulders relaxed.
2. Slowly bring your arms up above your head, with your palms facing each other. Fully extend your arms and lengthen your body upward, lifting your shoulders away from your ears.
3. Ensure that your body is aligned correctly, maintaining a straight and elongated spine. Activate your abdominal and core muscles to support your posture.

4. Inhaling deeply, bend your body forward from the pelvis, keeping your back straight and your arms stretched above your head. Bring your torso towards your thighs, trying to bring your chest closer to your legs.
5. Hold the position for a few deep, even breaths. Try to relax your head and neck, letting the weight of your head bring your entire body down. Keep your hands in contact with your body or the floor, depending on your flexibility level.
6. Feel the deep stretch in the hamstrings and back muscles. Breathe deeply, allowing your breath to further guide the stretch.
7. If you feel tension in your knees, you can bend them slightly to reduce the pressure on them.
8. As you exhale, gradually lift your torso to a standing position, raising your arms above your head. Return to the standing position, keeping your back straight and your arms extended.
9. You can repeat Hastha Uttanasana several times, concentrating on deep breathing and elongating your body with each repetition.

Hip opener stretch

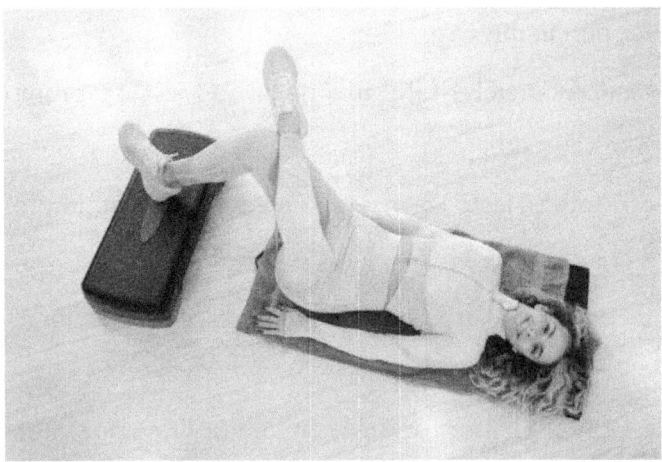

The Hip Opener Stretch is an exercise that aims to improve hip and glute flexibility.

Benefits:

- The exercise opens the hip joint, allowing for a greater range of motion and increasing flexibility in the area. This can be particularly beneficial for individuals who spend extended periods sitting, as it helps alleviate potential stiffness in the hips.
- Many people accumulate tension in the hip and buttock muscles due to a sedentary lifestyle or physical activities that involve these areas. The Hip Opener Stretch can help relax and release this tension, thus reducing any pain or discomfort.

- The hip and buttock muscles are essential for correct posture. Keeping these muscles flexible and healthy can help improve body alignment and prevent postural problems that can cause pain or tightness in other parts of the body, such as the back.
- Having a flexible and well-functioning hip is important to prevent injuries during daily activities or sports. The Hip Opener Stretch can assist in enhancing hip mobility and mitigating the risk of injuries associated with muscle stiffness.
- Hip flexibility is closely linked to back health. Reducing tension and improving hip mobility through stretching can help relieve lower back pain associated with poor posture or limited muscle flexibility.

Execution:
1. Begin by sitting on the floor with your knees bent and your feet flat on the ground in front of you. Maintain a straight back and relax your arms at your sides.
2. Bring one foot over the opposite knee so that the ankle rests on top of the knee. Make sure your foot is still and your knee is slightly bent. The knee forms a 90-degree angle.
3. Inhaling, keep your back straight and slowly lean your torso forward towards your bent knee.
4. Strive to keep your back flat and your chest open. You can place your hands on the floor or on the opposite foot for support as needed.
5. Once you reach full extension, you may begin to feel an intense stretching sensation in the outside hip and buttock portion of the bent knee. Hold the position and take deep breaths, allowing the muscles to relax and gradually release.
6. Hold the position for 20-30 seconds, continuing to breathe deeply and relaxing into the movement. Try to keep muscle tension at a comfortable level, avoiding excessive force.
7. After completing the stretch on one side, switch legs and repeat the process on the other side. Be sure to maintain symmetry and stability while performing the exercise on both sides.
8. After performing the Hip Opener Stretch on both sides, you can relax by sitting on the floor and breathing deeply for a few breaths, allowing your muscles to relax completely.

Crescent Moon Pose

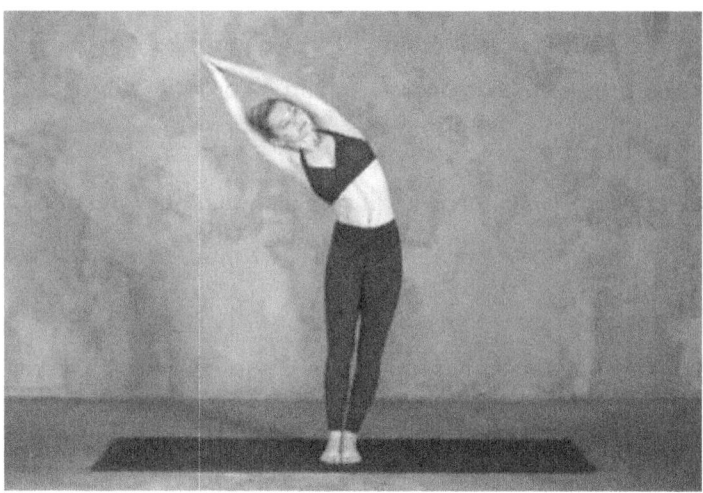

Crescent Moon Pose, also known as Ardha Chandrasana in Sanskrit, is a yoga pose that involves a sideways tilt of the body with one leg raised.

Benefits:

- The crescent helps to lengthen the lateral muscles of the trunk, promoting flexibility of the spine.
- To maintain balance in this position, it is necessary to activate the abdominal and core muscles, contributing to their strengthening.
- This position requires considerable balance and concentration, helping to improve both aspects.
- Raising a leg and holding the position requires stability and strength in the legs and feet, helping to improve the overall stability of the body.
- The crescent moon pose can stimulate the digestive and circulatory systems, improving the overall health of the internal organs.
- Leaning to the side and breathing deeply can help release built-up tension in your muscles and calm your mind.

Execution:

1. Start standing, with your feet together or slightly apart.
2. Place your weight on your left foot and bends your right knee, lifting right foot off the floor.
3. Bring both arms up above your head, fully extending them.
4. Tilt your torso to the left side, placing your body weight on your left foot, and extending your right arm towards the ceiling.
5. Lift your right leg while simultaneously keeping your body aligned, forming a straight line from the tips of your right toes to the tips of your right fingers.
6. Keep your neck in line with the spine, your gaze can be directed towards the thumb of the raised hand or upwards.

7. Maintain this position for a few deep breaths, then gradually return to the standing position.
8. Repeat on the opposite side, lifting your left leg and leaning towards the right side.

Exercises to calm nervous system

The nervous system plays an important role in regulating our responses to daily stress, tension, and agitation. Somatic exercises offer an effective approach to calming the nervous system, reducing activation of the sympathetic nervous system (responsible for the stress response), and promoting an overall sense of calm and tranquility.

Heaviness exercise

Heaviness exercise is a relaxation technique that aims to induce a state of calm and tranquility through deep muscle relaxation.

This type of practice can be particularly beneficial for addressing problems related to insomnia and promoting a general state of well-being.

Execution:

1. Make sure you are in a comfortable position, lying on a bed or on a comfortable surface. You can also perform the exercise in a sitting position, as long as your body is relaxed.
2. Start by focusing on your breathing. Breathe slowly and deeply, feeling the air move in and out of your body. This initial step helps you create a state of awareness and calm.
3. After reaching a state of calm through breathing, focus your attention on the part of the body you want to relax. It can be the left leg, for example.
4. Imagine that your left leg becomes heavy, very heavy. Visualize and experience the sensation of heaviness spreading through your leg muscles. Imagine that your body is anchored to the floor due to its excessive heaviness.
5. After experiencing heaviness in one part of the body, you can proceed to other areas such as the other leg, abdomen, arms and so on. Each time, imagine and feel the deep relaxation and feeling of heaviness.
6. You can also focus on your entire body, imagining your entire body becoming heavy and relaxed. Feel the weight of your body on the bed or surface you are lying on.
7. Repeat the heaviness exercise for a period that seems appropriate to you. It is helpful to practice regularly, preferably every day, to achieve maximum benefits. You can adjust the duration according to your needs and the available time.

Diaphragmatic breathing or abdominal breathing

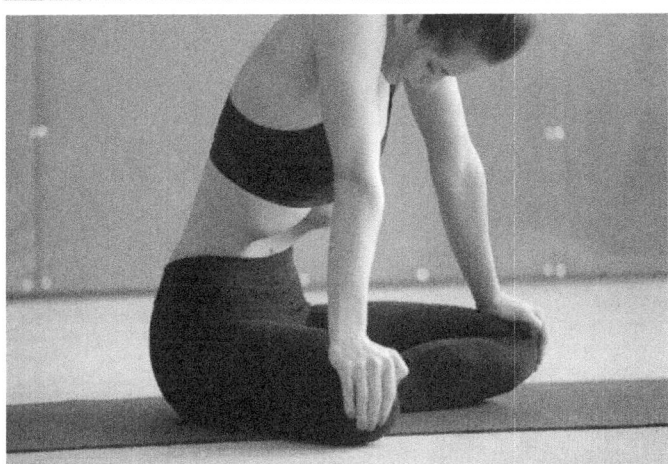

Breathing is the most important and at the same time the most natural gesture that we perform every day. Breathing allows the brain to function, metabolizes food, helps eliminate waste substances from the body and regenerates cells.

One might assume that since it is so important to breathe, everyone can do so.

Obviously, this is true, but it is equally true that not everyone knows how to breathe correctly.

Most people, in fact, breathe superficially, filling only a small part of their lungs with air and consequently living in a perpetual state of poor oxygenation, without being able to benefit from the many benefits of correct breathing. However, it is possible, in a simple and effective way, to return to breathing naturally, using the diaphragm as a cure to improve your physical and mental health.

Breathing with the diaphragm helps you move from the fight or flight state, in which the body is ready to react to a danger, to the rest and digest state, in which a sense of tranquility and relaxation prevails.

Execution:

1. Lie on your back on the floor or in bed or sit comfortably in a chair.
2. Place one hand on your chest and the other on your belly, just below your belly button. This allows you to feel the movement of your diaphragm as you breathe.
3. Inhale slowly through your nose and visualize the air descending directly into your belly as if it were inflating a balloon positioned at the height of your navel.
4. Feel your belly swelling under your hand, while the other hand positioned on your chest remains as still as possible.
5. When you exhale, open your mouth and let the air out passively without contracting your abdominal muscles or arching your back. Also, in this case the hand on the chest must remain still. The goal is: no movement of the chest, but only of the belly.

6. Breathe well in this way for at least 10 minutes, always remaining very focused on the correct execution of the exercise: inhale through your nose - inflate your belly - do not move your chest - exhale with your mouth wide open.
7. It's among the breathing methods that are highly effective in inducing relaxation. You can perform it in any posture, especially when you require a brief relaxation period. Initially, it's advisable to lie down with your hands gently resting on the abdomen beside the navel.
8. In the first tries, aim to gently encourage inhalation by expanding the belly outward and exhalation by contracting it (as if you're pulling the navel inward). With practice, this breathing pattern will become second nature to you.

The Ujjayi breath

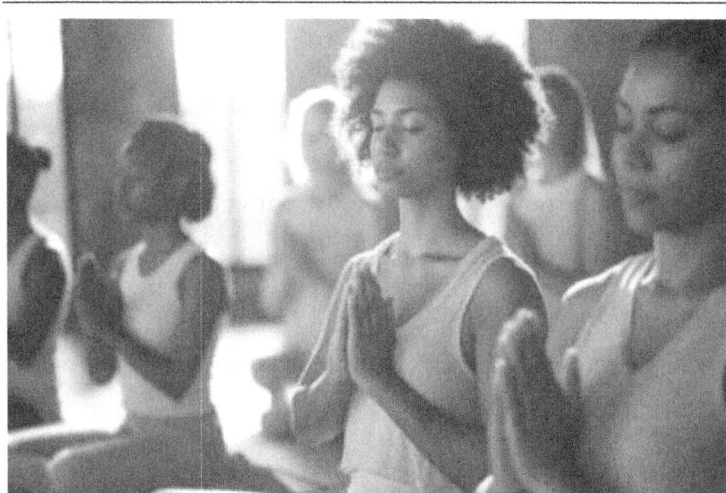

Ujjayi breath is widely utilized by practitioners worldwide because of its myriad advantages.

Benefits:

- It produces a warming effect that increases body temperature.
- The heart rate slows down and the circulatory system improves.
- By regulating your breath, your mind becomes tranquil, and you gain heightened awareness of your internal state.
- Unlike other Pranayama techniques that require practicing in a still, meditative position, this breathing technique can also be incorporated during the execution of yoga asanas.
- Deep breathing, in particular, enhances lung elasticity, resulting in overall benefits for the respiratory system.
- Through focusing on the sound of breathing, one can forge a connection between the mind, body, and spirit.
- It is especially advantageous for soothing the mind, alleviating stress, and diminishing any kind of nervous tension.

- It makes the gas exchanges that take place in the lungs more efficient.
- Its profound relaxation effect makes it an excellent remedy for combating insomnia.

Execution:

1. Find a comfortable position to sit or lie down. You can also stand if you prefer. Make sure you keep your spine straight and relaxed.
2. Begin to relax your body, paying attention to your shoulders, chest and abdomen. Relax completely but maintain an upright and mindful posture.
3. Start by inhaling slowly through your nose, allowing the air to deeply penetrate your lungs. While inhaling, concentrate on the sensation of filling your abdomen, ribs, and rib cage with air.
4. As you inhale, slightly contract the back of your throat. Imagine making the "ha-ha" sound as if you were fogging up a mirror with your breath, but not actually doing it. This contracting of the throat creates a slight restriction on airflow.
5. Exhalation: Slowly, exhale through your nose. As you exhale, contract your throat again as you did during the inhalation. This should create a soft, prolonged sound, like the sound of the sea.
6. Try to maintain a constant flow of breath, without significant pauses between inhalation and exhalation. The sound should be uniform and continuous.
7. Start by dedicating a few minutes each day to practicing this breathing technique. As you grow more accustomed to Ujjayi breathing, gradually increase the duration of your practice sessions.

Supta Baddha Konasana

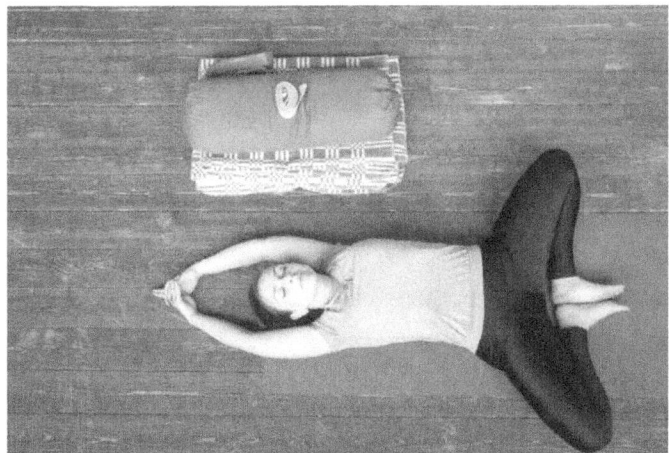

Supta Baddha Konasana is a yoga position that promotes a deep state of psychophysical relaxation. This position is always useful, especially when you need to distract yourself mentally and relax deeply. It is particularly suitable even in cases of strong tension and tiredness.

Although it is a simple pose, Supta Baddha Konasana is not recommended if you have pain or have had knee surgery. If the discomfort is slight, the position can be performed using a folded blanket or yoga bricks at the point below the knees.

Execution:

1. Sit on a yoga mat on the floor with the soles of your feet touching and your knees spreading outward. Place a pillow or a rolled blanket behind you, so that when you bring your back to the ground, the pillow remains between your shoulder blades, along the line of your spine, from the lumbar area to the nape of your neck.
2. As you exhale, gently lower your back toward the floor. If needed, you can rest your elbows on the ground for support if you feel unsure.
3. Your entire back must be completely stretched out on the ground and your sacrum and upper part of your buttocks must touch the mat well.
4. With your hands, grasp the upper inner part of your thighs and rotate them slightly outwards.
5. Slide your hands along the outside of your thighs towards your knees and spread your knees apart, trying to move them apart.
6. At this stage, position your hands on the floor at an angle of about 45 degrees from your torso, with your palms facing upward. Breathe and relax.
7. Try to maintain this position until you can balance both effort and relaxation.
8. Gradually release from the position. Utilize your hands to guide your thighs together, then gently roll to one side and slowly rise to a seated position.

Cat Cow Pose

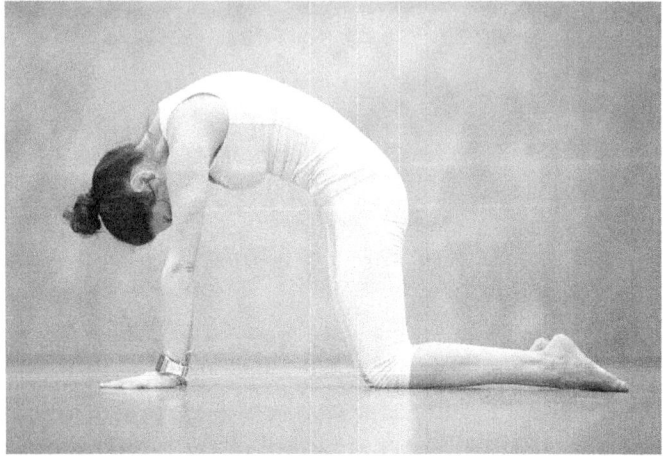

The sequence of Marjariasana (Cat Pose) and Bitilasana (Cow Pose) offers various benefits for the body and mind.

Benefits:

- The sequence incorporates flexion and extension movements of the spine, aiding in enhancing its flexibility and mobility.
- The Cat pose stretches the back muscles, while the Cow pose contracts them. This cycle helps strengthen your back muscles, improving stability and strength.
- Alternating flexion and extension movements can help stimulate internal organs, aid digestion and improve the function of abdominal organs.
- Coordination of the breath with the movements in this sequence promotes greater awareness of the breath.
- The practice of Marjariasana-Bitilasana can induce a calming effect on both the body and mind, assisting in alleviating accumulated stress and tension.
- Enhancing the strength of your back muscles and augmenting spinal flexibility can contribute to enhancing your overall posture.
- Extension and flexion poses can have calming effects on the nervous system, helping to relax the body and promote a sense of well-being.

Execution:

1. Begin by positioning yourself on a yoga mat, placing your hands and knees on the mat. Ensure your wrists are directly under your shoulders and your knees are positioned under your hips.
2. Start by performing the Cow Pose. Inhale and push your belly towards the mat, while simultaneously lifting your chin and opening your chest. You look up, arching your back downwards. You lower your shoulders, away from your ears.
3. Then, move to the Cat position. Exhale, arching your back upwards to make a hump, and withdraw your belly. Turn your head towards the floor, bringing your chin towards your chest. Relax your neck muscles and look at your thighs.
4. Inhale and return to Cow Pose. Then exhale again and repeat the Cat pose.
5. Repeat this sequence from 5 to 20 times depending on your needs.

Erected Pole (zhan zhuang)

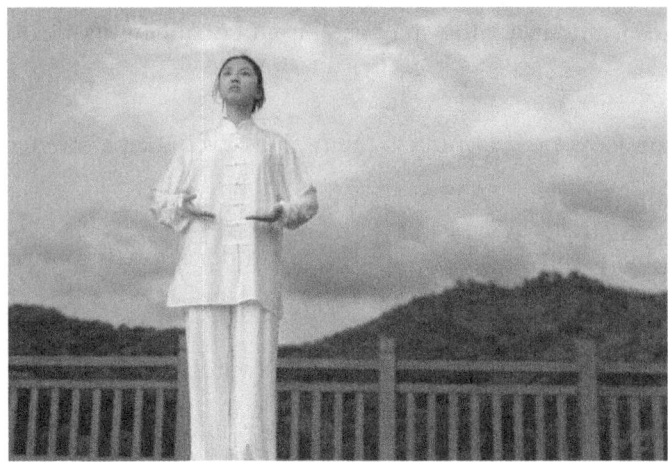

The Erect Pole also called "hugging the tree", is certainly the best-known type of static qi gong.

In fact, this Qi Gong consists of projecting deep roots into the ground from the center of the foot which allow the arms to rise naturally, without any effort, leaving the neck and shoulders free to listen to the energy that moves harmoniously or as may happen, that gets stuck in some muscle or joint.

Benefits:

- The practice helps strengthen and circulate internal energy (Qi) in the body. The static position allows you to focus attention on the accumulation and distribution of energy.
- The Erect Pole promotes energetic balance, harmonizing the Yin and Yang polarities in the body. This can lead to a greater feeling of well-being and stability.
- The upright position helps improve posture and strengthen the muscular structure. It can help prevent or alleviate problems related to poor posture.
- Maintaining the Upright Pole position requires constant muscular effort, helping to develop strength in the muscles of the legs, trunk and upper body.
- The practice of Qi Gong is known for its relaxing effects. The Erect Pole, in particular, can help reduce stress, promoting a calmer mental state.
- The static position requires intense concentration on the experience of the present moment. This can promote greater mental clarity and concentration.
- Regular practice can have positive effects on sleep quality, helping to reduce insomnia and promote deeper rest.

Execution:

1. Stand with your feet facing forward, parallel to each other, and firmly planted on the ground shoulder-width apart. Sink your feet into the ground, keeping them elastic, with the tips of your toes slightly extended.
2. Extend your body upward, elongating the spine and stretching the top of your head toward the sky. Aim for the sensation that your head is floating effortlessly above your neck, suspended gracefully above your spine.

3. Gently push your hips forward, as though you're perched on the edge of a tall stool. This adjustment will straighten the spine in the lower back, as many people have a natural "s" curve in the spine. The primary goal of this standing position is to minimize the curvature of the spine to facilitate the smooth flow of energy.
4. Maintain a slight bend in your knees. Avoid locking your knees, ensuring they are never overly straight, and be cautious not to allow them to extend past your toes.
5. Relax your shoulders, avoiding excessive arching of the back as in a military stance. Instead, aim to create a slight curve in the upper part of your back, allowing your chest to gently concave.
6. Let your arms rest comfortably at the sides of your body. Keep your hands and arms relaxed and free, as they hang at your sides.
7. Let your palms face your hips. Because of the small space under your armpits, your hands will not touch your hips, but will hang about 4 or 5 centimeters away.
8. Bring your chin back slightly as you push up towards the top of your head. This gesture opens the area where the spine meets the skull.
9. Keep your eyes half closed looking straight ahead. Maintaining your eyes partially open can help avoid distractions, while closing them completely may induce tiredness and drowsiness. A relaxed gaze with half-closed eyes provides optimal conditions for effective meditation.
10. Gently place your tongue on the roof of your mouth, keeping your lips parted. Relax your jaw muscles.
11. I recommend that you focus on one or two alignment points at a time, adding the next ones only when you feel ready.

Conscious breathing

Mindful breathing, or mindfulness breathing, is a practice that involves conscious attention on the breath.

Benefits:

- Mindful breathing serves as a valuable tool for managing stress and anxiety. Concentrating on your breath can effectively quiet the mind, diminish stress levels, and foster a sense of tranquility.
- The practice of mindful breathing requires a focus on the act of breathing. This can train the mind to focus on a single item, improving concentration and attention.
- Mindful breathing can help regulate emotions. Practicing breath awareness can be an effective way to manage intense emotions, allowing for a more balanced response to events.
- The practice of mindful breathing can promote relaxation and help improve the quality of sleep. Slow, deep breathing aids in reducing activation of the sympathetic nervous system, thereby preparing the body for rest and relaxation.

- Breath awareness can help relax muscle tension in the body. Often, during times of stress, people can develop muscle tension, and conscious breathing can help release this tension.
- Regular practice of mindful breathing can increase body awareness. This means being more aware of physical sensations and the body's reactions, which can be useful for managing pain or preventing habitual behaviors that are harmful to your health.

Execution

1. It is an exercise that can be done standing or sitting, anywhere and at any time. All you have to do is stay still and focus on your breathing for just one minute.
2. Start breathing and exhale slowly. One breathing cycle should last approximately 6 seconds. Inhale through your nose and expel the air through your mouth, letting your breath flow effortlessly, in and out of your body.
3. Letting go of your thoughts for a minute. You don't think about the things you still have to do today, and you don't reflect on your life plans. Simply let yourself go for a minute without thinking about anything except your breathing.
4. Concentrate on breathing with particular attention. Notice the sensation of the air entering the body and filling you with life, follow its path to your mouth and feel the energy dissipating into the world.
5. And if you think you are not able to meditate, you should know that with this exercise you are already halfway there. If you have felt better, relaxed, calm and recharged, try increasing the time from one to five minutes gradually, you will benefit from the long-term effects of this calming practice.

The position of intoxicating bliss

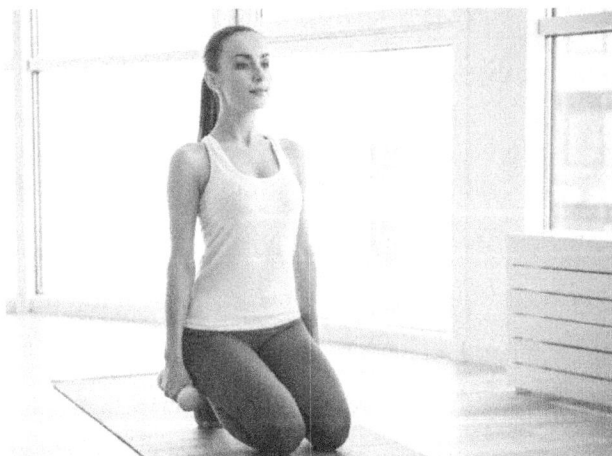

The Ananda Madirasana yoga position is a practice that brings numerous physical and mental benefits.

Benefits:

- Through regular practice of this yoga position, you can achieve a state of mental calm and tranquility, helping to reduce stress and nervous system agitation.

- The position can promote blood flow in the abdomen, thus stimulating the digestive system and helping to improve digestion.
- Some movements and pressures resulting from the practice of Ananda Madirasana can promote the well-being and balance of the reproductive system.
- By focusing attention and concentration during practice, you can cultivate a heightened awareness of your body and its movements.
- The position promotes bodily alignment which leads to a sense of internal balance and a feeling of calm and tranquility.
- Due to its ability to soothe both the mind and body, Ananda Madirasana can be beneficial in alleviating emotional stress and anxiety.

Execution:
1. Begin by assuming a seated position on the yoga mat. Extend your legs in front of you, ensuring your back is straight.
2. Flex your left knee and place your left heel near your left buttock, keeping your knee bent on the ground.
3. Take your right foot and position it on top of your left thigh, near your bent left knee. Make sure your right foot is positioned well and your right knee is open outward.
4. Extend your right arm behind you and place it on the floor near your right buttock. Use your right arm as support to maintain balance as you rotate your torso to the right.
5. Flex your left arm and bring it above your right knee. Place your left elbow on the outside of your right knee, then raise your left hand up, forming a prayer position.
6. Once in the full Ananda Madirasana position, hold the position for a few deep, slow breaths. Concentrate on your breathing and try to relax your mind and body.
7. After holding the position for an appropriate amount of time, slowly release the position and repeat the process on the opposite side, bending your right leg and rotating your torso to the left.
8. After completing both sides, return to a sitting position and take a few deep breaths before finishing the practice.

Exercises to relieve chronic pain

Chronic pain can deeply affect an individual's quality of life, constraining their capacity to engage in daily activities and leading to both physical and emotional distress. Somatic exercises offer an integrated and mindful approach to alleviating chronic pain, engaging the mind and body to promote muscle relaxation, improve posture and reduce the activation of the nervous system responsible for pain perception.

Pelvic Clock

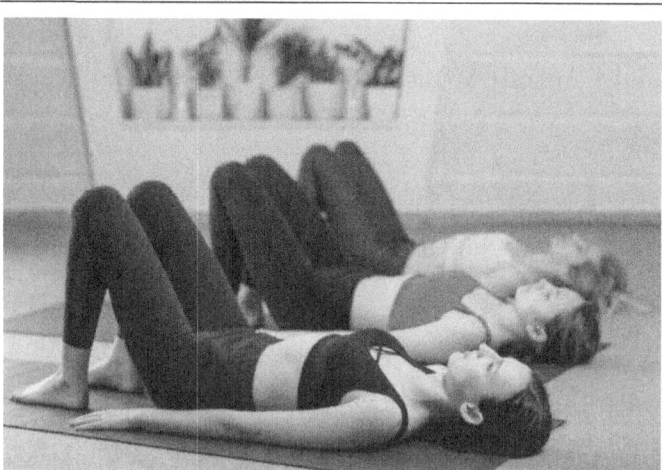

The pelvic clock exercise is a key concept in Somatic Exercises, which focuses on awareness and control of pelvic movements.

Benefits:

- This exercise can help improve your mind-body connection and reduce tension in your lower back.
- The ability to correctly perform a pelvic tilt will have positive effects on the execution of the squat and deadlift, improving flexibility, facilitating more complex movements and contributing to a deeper understanding of these exercises.
- The pelvic clock is a useful tool for developing awareness of the positioning of the abdominal, pelvis and spine. By performing this controlled movement, you can focus on specific activation of the abdominal and pelvic floor muscles, helping to improve coordination and alignment of the body.
- This type of exercise can be useful in improving flexibility, stability and body awareness, thus reducing any tension and contributing to the relief of chronic pain in the lower back and pelvic area.
- During pregnancy, the pelvic clock exercise can be a useful resource for maintaining pelvic mobility and stability. It can also be part of prenatal or postpartum exercise programs to help maintain pelvic floor strength and health. For pregnant women, exercise can help relieve back pain by promoting posture awareness and strengthening the lumbar and pelvic muscles.

Execution:

1. Lie on your back on a mat, with your knees bent and feet flat on the ground, ensuring they're parallel to the ground. Maintain a relaxed and neutral spine position. Relax your neck and shoulders, gently moving your shoulders away from your ears.
2. Join your hands together so that the tips of your index fingers and thumbs touch each other.
3. Now place your hands on the lower part of your abdomen, so that your fingertips are positioned above your pubic bone while your thumbs are pointing and positioned near your navel.
4. Inhale deeply, evenly expanding your ribs and engaging your lower abdominal as well.
5. Engage your abs and lower your lower abdomen toward your spine, extending your spine along the floor. This will create a pelvic tilt where your watch is now no longer flat but tilted downwards at the 12 o'clock position and upwards at the 6 o'clock position.
6. Use your abs to rotate the clock sideways so that your 3 o'clock hip is lower. Continue to inhale, moving your pelvis through the 24-hour cycle, tilting until the 6 o'clock position becomes your lowest.
7. Continuing the movement, lower the hip to 9 o'clock. Continue exhaling and bring the umbilical part back to the lowest point.
8. Repeat the exact same cycle on the other side of your body. Perform three sets of repetitions on each side, totaling six sets in all.

Cross twist position

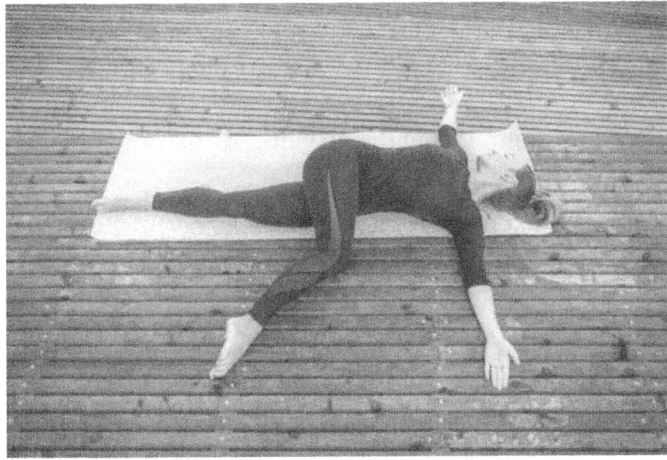

Supta Matsyendrasana, or supine spinal cross twist pose, is a yoga pose that involves twisting the spine while lying on your back.

Benefits:

- Twisting the spine in Supta Matsyendrasana can aid in relaxing and elongating the muscles of the lower back, which may help alleviate pain and enhance flexibility.

- The twists stimulate the digestive system, promoting better circulation and stimulation of the abdominal organs. This practice can aid in improving digestion and alleviating gastrointestinal issues.
- The pose can be used as a warm-up, preparing the spine for more intense poses involving backbends. This helps improve spinal flexibility and reduce the risk of injury.
- The twist and relaxation offered by Supta Matsyendrasana can help relieve pain and cramps during the menstrual cycle by improving circulation in the abdominal area and relaxing the muscles.
- You can practice this asana at night to promote better sleep. Perform it gently and synchronize your breathing throughout the movement for optimal results.

Execution:

1. Lie on your back on a yoga mat or any soft surface, extending your legs straight and allowing your arms to rest in a relaxed position by your sides.
2. Take a deep breath, relax, and come into reclining mountain pose. Ensure that your neck, spine, and shoulders remain flat on the floor.
3. Inhale gently and deeply, then bend your left leg (left knee), bringing it closer to your chest. Allow your knees to bend and relax in this pose for about 2 to 3 breaths.
4. Now, for the twist, exhale and guide your left (bent) knee towards the right side of your body. Rotate your hips and position them at the center of your body on the mat, with your left knee touching the floor (if your knee doesn't touch the mat, that's okay).
5. Shift your hips slightly to the left. Your left hip should be resting on your right thigh.
6. Ensure that your shoulder blades are touching the ground and extend your right arm in line with your shoulder, with the palm facing down.
7. The left hand can be extended (forming both arms) with the palm facing the ground, or you can hold it above the bent left knee.
8. Turn your head to the left and stare at the fingertips of your left hand.
9. Keep your extended leg straight.
10. Remain in this supine twist position and take relaxed breaths, inhaling and exhaling deeply. Release all stress and tension from your body with each breath.
11. When you're ready to release, bring your head back to the center, lower your left leg to the ground, and extend it fully.
12. Now relax and do it on the other side with your right leg.

Garland Pose

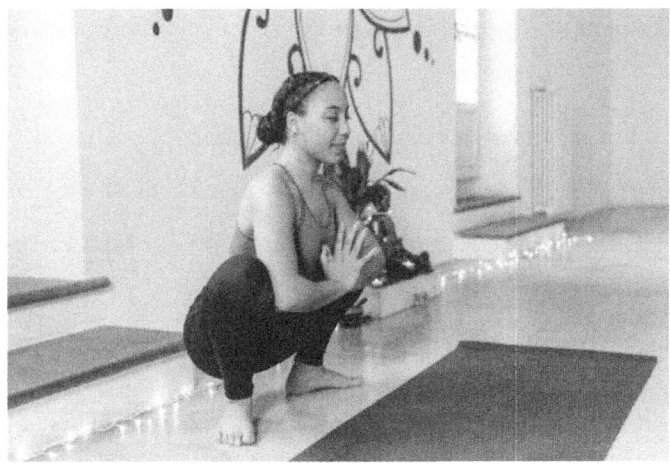

The Garland Pose, also called Malasana, is a yoga position that offers various benefits to combat pain, especially in the lower back, hips and knees.

Benefits:

- Malasana actively engages the leg muscles, including the quadriceps, hamstrings, and calf muscles. This can help strengthen and tone these muscle areas, reducing the load on the lower back and relieving associated pain.
- Malasana stretches and opens the hip muscles, including the hip flexors and adductor muscles. This can help improve hip flexibility and mobility, reducing pressure on your lower back and hips.
- Garland Pose involves a gentle lengthening of the spine, helping to reduce compression and tension in the lower back. This can help relieve chronic or acute lower back pain.
- Malasana can aid in improving posture, particularly beneficial for individuals who spend extended periods sitting or standing. Lengthening the spine and strengthening the muscles of the legs and buttocks can promote a more upright and balanced posture, reducing the risk of back and hip pain.
- The practice of Malasana, along with deep, mindful breathing, can help reduce stress and anxiety, which are often related to chronic pain. The relaxing and meditative position can promote a feeling of calm and mental well-being.

Execution:

1. Begin by standing with your feet slightly wider than your hips and angled slightly outward, approximately 45 degrees. Keep your arms resting at your sides.
2. Bend your knees slightly and tilt your torso forward, bringing your hands to the center of your chest in a prayer position.
3. Bring your knees outward, keeping your feet on the floor. Try to bring your thighs as close to the floor as possible.

4. Slowly lower your pelvis down, keeping your knees bent and pushed outward. Try to keep your weight on your heels to maintain balance.
5. As you lower your hips, bring your arms inside your knees, with your elbows slightly bent.
6. The hands should be clasped together in a prayerful gesture, with the palms firmly pressed against each other.
7. Use your elbows to push slightly outward on your knees, creating an additional stretch in your hips and groin area.
8. Hold for a few deep, even breaths, focusing on relaxing your shoulders and neck. Try to maintain smooth, continuous breathing.
9. Ensure to maintain a straight back throughout the pose. Avoid collapsing your chest forward but try to keep your chest lifted.
10. To come out of the position, slowly lift your pelvis upward, extending your legs and returning to standing. Breathe deeply and move slowly to avoid dizziness.

Swan dive

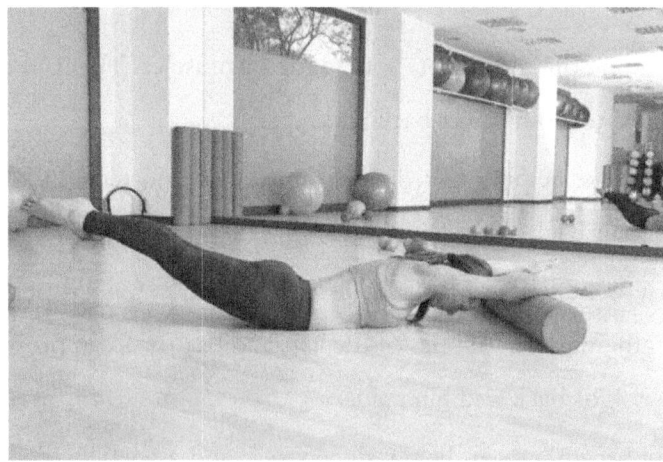

The Swan Dive is a Pilates exercise that can offer several benefits for relieving pain, particularly in the case of back pain.

Benefits:

- The Swan Dive involves a wide range of spinal movements, from extension to flexion, which can help improve spinal flexibility.
- During the Swan Dive, you use your core and upper body muscles to lift your chest off the floor. This aids in strengthening your back muscles, enhancing stability, and minimizing the risk of injury.
- The Swan Dive also involves the shoulder and triceps muscles, promoting the extension and relaxation of these joints. This can help reduce tension and pain in the shoulder and neck area.

- The Swan Dive, like many Pilates exercises, encourages concentration and relaxation through controlled breathing and fluid movement. This can help in diminishing both mental and physical stress and tension, which may be associated with chronic pain.

Execution:

1. Begin by lying on your stomach on the mat, extending your legs behind you and spreading your feet the width of the mat. Your arms should be extended at your sides with the palms of your hands facing down.
2. Make sure your upper legs and pelvis are on the ground and your spine is in a neutral position. Activate your core muscles by gently squeezing them to stabilize your pelvis and lower back.
3. Inhale as you gradually lift your torso off the floor, maintaining straight arms at your sides. Maintain a slight bend in your elbows and bring your shoulders back and down, lengthening the front of your body.
4. Continue lifting your torso while simultaneously raising your legs off the floor.
5. Use your leg and glute muscles to lift your legs as high as possible, keeping your knees slightly bent.
6. Once you're completely off the floor, form an "U" with your body, with your torso and legs raised as high as possible. Hold this position for a deep breath, feeling the lengthening of your spine and engaging your core muscles.
7. Exhale as you slowly lower your torso and legs to the floor, returning to the starting position. Maintain control of the movement and make sure you maintain good posture as you return to the starting position.

Chapter 9: 30-days Somatic Exercises Challenge

Welcome to the 30-Day Somatic Exercise Challenge! This challenge will take you through a series of exercises designed to improve your body awareness, release built-up tension and promote overall well-being of body and mind.

During this challenge, we will explore a wide range of somatic exercises, including yoga poses, mindful breathing, stretching, and fluid movements. Every day you will have a new set of exercises to complete. Remember that the main goal of this challenge is not only to complete the exercises, but also to be aware of the sensations in your body as you perform them. Take the time to listen to your body, adjust exercises to your needs, and practice self-kindness along the way.

Day 1:

1. Utkatasana (Chair Pose) - Hold for 30 seconds, repeat 3 times with 10 second rest breaks between repetitions.
2. Bhujangasana (Cobra Pose) - Hold for 20 seconds, repeat 3 times with 10 second rest breaks between repetitions.
3. Boat Pose - Hold for 20 seconds, repeat 3 times with 10 second rest pauses between repetitions.

Day 2:

1. Hip Circles - Perform 10 circles clockwise and 10 counterclockwise for each leg.
2. Leg Circles - Perform 10 clockwise and 10 counterclockwise circles for each leg.
3. Child Pose - Hold for 30 seconds, repeat 3 times with 10 second rest pauses between repetitions.

Day 3:

1. Legs to the wall - Hold for 30 seconds, repeat 3 times with 10 second rest breaks between repetitions.
2. Box Breathing - Perform 3 full cycles of box breathing (4 seconds inhale, 4 seconds hold, 4 seconds exhale, 4 seconds pause).
3. Relaxing circle exercise - Perform 10 repetitions on each side.

Day 4:

1. Tree Pose - Hold for 30 seconds on each side, repeat 3 times with 10 second rest breaks between repetitions.
2. The movement of the Flowing River - Perform 10 repetitions.

3. The 5-4-3-2-1 Grounding Technique - Perform for 3 minutes.

Day 5:
1. Butterfly hug - Perform 10 butterfly hugs.
2. Fish Pose - Hold for 20 seconds, repeat 3 times with 10 second rest pauses between repetitions.
3. Corpse Pose - Relax in a supine position for 5 minutes, focusing on deep, relaxed breathing.

Day 6:
1. Forward Fold - Hold for 30 seconds, repeat 3 times with 10 second rest breaks between repetitions.
2. Eagle Pose - Hold for 20 seconds on each side, repeat 3 times with 10 second rest breaks between repetitions.
3. Hip Circles - Perform 10 circles clockwise and 10 counterclockwise for each leg.

Day 7:
1. Cow Pose - Hold for 30 seconds, repeat 3 times with 10 second rest breaks between repetitions.
2. Spine Stretch Forward - Hold for 20 seconds, repeat 3 times with 10 second rest breaks between repetitions.
3. Arm Swings - Perform 20 back and forth arm swings.

Day 8:
1. Raised arm Pose - Hold for 30 seconds, repeat 3 times with 10 second rest breaks between repetitions.
2. Hip opener stretch - Hold for 20 seconds on each side, repeat 3 times with 10 second rest breaks between repetitions.
3. Mermaid - Hold for 30 seconds each side, repeat 3 times with 10 second rest breaks between repetitions.

Day 9:
1. Mountain Pose - Hold for 30 seconds, repeat 3 times with 10 second rest pauses between repetitions.
2. Crescent Moon Pose - Hold for 20 seconds on each side, repeat 3 times with 10 second rest breaks between repetitions.
3. The Saw - Perform 10 repetitions.

Day 10:
1. Diaphragmatic breathing or abdominal breathing - Perform for 5 minutes, focusing on deep, controlled breathing.
2. Supta Baddha Konasana - Hold for 30 seconds, repeat 3 times with 10 second rest breaks between repetitions.

3. Cat Cow Pose - Perform 10 repetitions, alternating between cat and cow pose.

Day 11:
1. Legs to the wall - Hold for 30 seconds, repeat 3 times with 10 second rest breaks between repetitions.
2. Feldenkrais Thoracic rotation - Perform 10 repetitions on each side.
3. Hip opener stretch - Hold for 20 seconds on each side, repeat 3 times with 10 second rest breaks between repetitions.

Day 12:
1. Child Pose - Hold for 30 seconds, repeat 3 times with 10 second rest pauses between repetitions.
2. Butterfly hug - Perform 10 butterfly hugs.
3. Spine Stretch Forward - Hold for 20 seconds, repeat 3 times with 10 second rest breaks between repetitions.

Day 13:
1. Single Leg Stretch - Perform 10 reps per side.
2. Cross twist position - Hold for 30 seconds on each side, repeat 3 times with 10 second rest breaks between repetitions.
3. Raised arm Pose - Hold for 20 seconds, repeat 3 times with 10 second rest breaks between repetitions.

Day 14:
1. Eagle Pose - Hold for 30 seconds on each side, repeat 3 times with 10 second rest breaks between repetitions.
2. Swan dive - Perform 10 repetitions.
3. Boat Pose - Hold for 20 seconds, repeat 3 times with 10 second rest pauses between repetitions.

Day 15:
1. Mountain Pose - Hold for 30 seconds, repeat 3 times with 10 second rest pauses between repetitions.
2. Garland Pose - Hold for 20 seconds, repeat 3 times with 10 second rest pauses between repetitions.
3. Heaviness exercise - Perform for 5 minutes, focusing on the feeling of heaviness and relaxation of the muscles.

Day 16:
1. Corpse Pose - Relax in a supine position for 5 minutes, focusing on deep, relaxed breathing.
2. Eagle Pose - Hold for 30 seconds on each side, repeat 3 times with 10 second rest breaks between repetitions.
3. Hip Circles - Perform 10 circles clockwise and 10 counterclockwise for each leg.

Day 17:
1. Forward Fold - Hold for 30 seconds, repeat 3 times with 10 second rest breaks between repetitions.
2. Fish Pose - Hold for 30 seconds, repeat 3 times with 10 second rest pauses between repetitions.
3. Box Breathing - Perform 3 complete cycles of box breathing (4 seconds inhale, 4 seconds hold, 4 seconds exhale, 4 seconds pause).

Day 18:
1. Mountain Pose - Hold for 30 seconds, repeat 3 times with 10 second rest pauses between repetitions.
2. Raised arm Pose - Hold for 30 seconds, repeat 3 times with 10 second rest breaks between repetitions.
3. Diaphragmatic breathing or abdominal breathing - Perform for 5 minutes, focusing on deep, controlled breathing.

Day 19:
1. Leg Circles - Perform 10 clockwise and 10 counterclockwise circles for each leg.
2. Spine Stretch Forward - Hold for 30 seconds, repeat 3 times with 10 second rest breaks between repetitions.
3. The movement of the Flowing River - Perform 10 repetitions.

Day 20:
1. Tree Pose - Hold for 30 seconds on each side, repeat 3 times with 10 second rest breaks between repetitions.
2. Cow Pose - Hold for 30 seconds, repeat 3 times with 10 second rest breaks between repetitions.
3. Relaxing circle exercise - Perform 10 repetitions on each side.

Day 21:
1. Butterfly Hug - Perform 10 butterfly hugs.
2. Mountain Pose - Hold for 30 seconds, repeat 3 times with 10 second rest pauses between repetitions.
3. Eagle Pose - Hold for 30 seconds on each side, repeat 3 times with 10 second rest breaks between repetitions.

Day 22:
1. Hip Opener Stretch - Hold for 30 seconds each side, repeat 3 times with 10 second rest breaks between repetitions.
2. Box Breathing - Perform 3 complete cycles of box breathing (4 seconds inhale, 4 seconds hold, 4 seconds exhale, 4 seconds pause).

3. Leg Circles - Perform 10 clockwise and 10 counterclockwise circles for each leg.

Day 23:
1. Relaxing Circle Exercise - Perform 10 repetitions on each side.
2. Raised Arm Pose - Hold for 30 seconds, repeat 3 times with 10 second rest pauses between repetitions.
3. The Saw - Perform 10 repetitions.

Day 24:
1. Child Pose - Hold for 30 seconds, repeat 3 times with 10 second rest pauses between repetitions.
2. Fish Pose - Hold for 30 seconds, repeat 3 times with 10 second rest pauses between repetitions.
3. Diaphragmatic Breathing or Abdominal Breathing - Perform for 5 minutes, focusing on deep, controlled breathing.

Day 25:
1. Legs to the Wall - Hold for 30 seconds, repeat 3 times with 10 second rest breaks between repetitions.
2. Spine Stretch Forward - Hold for 30 seconds, repeat 3 times with 10 second rest breaks between repetitions.
3. Corpse Pose - Relax in a supine position for 5 minutes, focusing on deep, relaxed breathing.

Day 26:
1. Boat Pose - Hold for 30 seconds, repeat 3 times with 10 second rest breaks between repetitions.
2. Hip Circles - Perform 10 circles clockwise and 10 counterclockwise for each leg.
3. Tree Pose - Hold for 30 seconds on each side, repeat 3 times with 10 second rest breaks between repetitions.

Day 27:
1. Utkatasana (Chair Pose) - Hold for 30 seconds, repeat 3 times with 10 second rest breaks between repetitions.
2. Feldenkrais Thoracic Rotation - Perform 10 repetitions per side.
3. Cross Twist Position - Hold for 30 seconds on each side, repeat 3 times with 10 second rest breaks between repetitions.

Day 28:
1. Raised Arm Pose - Hold for 30 seconds, repeat 3 times with 10 second rest pauses between repetitions.
2. Butterfly Hug - Perform 10 butterfly hugs.

3. Hip Opener Stretch - Hold for 30 seconds each side, repeat 3 times with 10 second rest breaks between repetitions.

Day 29:

1. Mountain Pose - Hold for 30 seconds, repeat 3 times with 10 second rest pauses between repetitions.
2. Forward Fold - Hold for 30 seconds, repeat 3 times with 10 second rest breaks between repetitions.
3. Swan Dive - Perform 10 repetitions.

Day 30:

1. Fish Pose - Hold for 30 seconds, repeat 3 times with 10 second rest pauses between repetitions.
2. Corpse Pose - Relax in a supine position for 5 minutes, focusing on deep, relaxed breathing.
3. Diaphragmatic Breathing or Abdominal Breathing - Perform for 5 minutes, focusing on deep, controlled breathing.

Conclusions

As you have observed in this book, somatic exercises provide a comprehensive method for enhancing overall physical, mental, and emotional wellness. Through movement awareness and mind-body integration, you can reduce chronic pain, improve posture and increase flexibility. Consistent practice of these exercises can lead to greater body awareness and better stress management. It is important to engage in a journey of self-exploration and personal growth to fully experience the benefits of somatic exercises. Whether it's for pain management, improved athletic performance, or simply general well-being, somatic exercises offer a valuable opportunity to connect with your body and live a more balanced and fulfilling life.

In summary, somatic exercises serve as a potent instrument for enhancing overall health and well-being through consistent and dedicated practice. Through movement awareness and mind-body integration, it is possible to achieve a series of tangible and lasting benefits. Furthermore, the deep connection with one's body promotes a sense of emotional and mental balance, thus enhancing the overall quality of life. In an increasingly fast-paced and stressful world, somatic exercises offer a refuge of calm and self-exploration, allowing individuals to discover and cultivate their inner vitality. Experiencing the benefits of these exercises requires discipline and patience, but the results that can be achieved are vastly rewarding, promoting lasting harmony between body, mind and spirit.

Do Not Go Yet; One Last Thing To Do

If you enjoyed this book or found it useful, I'd be very grateful if you'd post a short review on Amazon. Your support does make a difference, and I read all the reviews personally so I can get your feedback and make this book even better.

Thanks again for your support!

Made in the USA
Las Vegas, NV
25 June 2024

91494649R00046